ZERO SUGAR ONE MONTH

ZERO SUGAR ONE MONTH

REDUCE CRAVINGS - RESET METABOLISM
LOSE WEIGHT - CONTROL BLOOD SUGAR

A program to inspire and teach that locks in your focus, breaks patterned thinking, builds confidence, and motivates you to reach your sugar-free goal like never before.

DR. BECKY GILLASPY

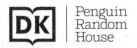

Penguin Random House

Publisher Mike Sanders
Editorial Director Ann Barton
Editor Brandon Buechley
Art Director William Thomas
Copy Editor Christopher Stolle
Cover Designer Lissa Auciello-Brogan
Compositor Ayanna Lacey
Proofreader Mira S. Park
Indexer Celia McCoy

First American Edition, 2023
Published in the United States by DK Publishing
1745 Broadway, 20th Floor, New York, NY 10019

The authorized representative in the EEA is Dorling Kindersley
Verlag GmbH. Arnulfstr. 124, 80636 Munich, Germany

Library of Congress Catalog Number: 2023941692
ISBN 978-0-7440-9482-4

Note: This publication is released with the understanding that the
author and publisher are not rendering professional services.
Consult your doctor before starting this program. Any change in
diet can impact aspects of your health, such as blood sugar levels,
medications, and other factors unique to you. If you feel unwell at
any time, stop the program and tell your doctor about the
symptoms you're experiencing.

DK books are available at special discounts when purchased in bulk
for sales promotions, premiums, fundraising, or educational use.
For details, contact: SpecialSales@dk.com

Printed and bound in the UK

www.dk.com

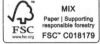

MIX
Paper | Supporting
responsible forestry
FSC™ C018179

This book was made with Forest
Stewardship Council ™ certified
paper – one small step in DK's
commitment to a sustainable future.
For more information go to
www.dk.com/our-green-pledge

To Keith, my husband and best friend.

CONTENTS

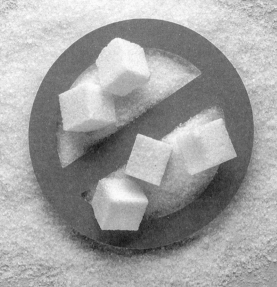

PART ONE
HOW TO BE
SUGAR-FREE

WELCOME TO YOUR SUGAR-FREE MONTH! YOU'RE IN THE RIGHT PLACE.

Sugar is the great deceiver. It gives you a quick energy burst and takes the edge off of everyday stressors. But you can't outrun the consequences of a high-sugar diet. Its addictive draw and inflammatory impact will lead to weight gain and contribute to heart disease, memory decline, bowel disorders, and other chronic conditions.

It is clear that eating sugar causes problems. But that knowledge does little to prevent us from wanting to eat it. Removing sugar from your diet requires action, and that requires motivation and a new perspective. This 30-day handbook gives you those necessary elements.

The goal of *Zero Sugar / One Month* is to eliminate added sugar from your diet for 30 consecutive days.

Suitable for any dietary preference from keto to vegetarian, this user-friendly handbook provides quick-reference guides that share the ground rules, what to eat when sugar is off the table, how to temptation-proof your life, and a timeline of what to expect.

Each day offers timely tips, targeted action steps, and fun and inspiring messages to guide you through emotional ups and downs, build your confidence, and keep you moving forward one day at a time.

Without sugar assaulting your tastebuds, you'll enjoy the subtle sweetness of whole foods, finding sugary treats too sweet. You'll reduce inflammation in your body, leading to clearer skin, fewer bathroom issues, and more energy.

Whenever you decide to start a healthy journey, the timing will seem off. Your mind will come up with many reasons to put things off till tomorrow. The unfortunate fact is that tomorrow never comes, but time passes. So, the question is, "Where do I want to be next month?" It only takes 30 days. You can do this!

HOW TO USE THIS BOOK

At its heart, *Zero Sugar / One Month* is a daily guide to keep you motivated and engaged during your 30-day sugar-free journey. On page 15, you'll find the ground rules, so you are clear on what exactly it means to be sugar-free. You'll then move into the "Day 0 Prep" section that provides the planning resources you'll use to set yourself up for success. When you're prepped and ready to go, you'll start your *Zero Sugar* month with Day 1.

Each day is broken down into four sections, based on a simple formula:

Focus + Motivation + Action = Results

I recommend reading each daily guide first thing in the morning, but if that doesn't fit your lifestyle, you can read them at the end of the day to prepare for tomorrow.

Daily Focus: This brief statement acts as a memory jogger. Carry *Zero Sugar / One Month* with you, and when sugar taps on your shoulder trying to get your attention, open the book and quickly reengage by rereading the daily focus.

Daily Motivation: Motivation is not something you go out and find somewhere ... out there. Quite the opposite. True motivation lives inside of you. You just need something to pull it to the surface. The daily motivation section does that for you using fun and inspirational stories and dialogues. Why the stories? Stories stick with you. Your mind returns to a story more than a rule or an assertion. They strengthen your resolve and reassure you that the experience you are having is normal and expected.

Daily Action: The overarching goal of the program is to avoid added sugar for 30 consecutive days. In addition, you will be given daily action steps. Think of them as the homework assignments that help you get a perfect grade on your "I Did It!" Report Card. While most of the daily actions can be completed in a few minutes, they will form the building blocks you need to cement your new healthy habits.

Daily Result and Reflections: At the end of each day, you'll get the opportunity to put a check mark in your "I Did It!" Report Card, celebrating the completion of one more glorious sugar-free day. This section also provides you with prompts and space to record your thoughts about the day. This self-reflection exercise is optional but will enhance your experience and solidify your results.

Many days also include stories from individuals who have followed a no-sugar path to success. You'll learn just how some of these focuses, motivations, and actions have benefited others, helping chart the course forward for your own success.

ZERO SUGAR / ONE MONTH "I DID IT!" REPORT CARD

There is nothing more motivating than being able to say, *"I did it!"* Below is your daily "I Did It!" Report Card.

DAY 1	DAY 2	DAY 3	DAY 4	DAY 5	DAY 6	DAY 7
DAY 8	**DAY 9**	**DAY 10**	**DAY 11**	**DAY 12**	**DAY 13**	**DAY 14**
DAY 15	**DAY 16**	**DAY 17**	**DAY 18**	**DAY 19**	**DAY 20**	**DAY 21**
DAY 22	**DAY 23**	**DAY 24**	**DAY 25**	**DAY 26**	**DAY 27**	**DAY 28**
DAY 29	**DAY 30**					

**CONGRATULATIONS!
YOU DID IT!**

How to Complete Your "I Did It!" Report Card: At the end of each successful no-sugar day, you'll acknowledge your accomplishment by placing a mark in the corresponding box.

That pat on the back can be a simple check mark, but keep in mind that this is a celebration! There is nothing wrong with drawing a smiley face, writing the word *"YAY,"* or pressing on a daily sticker. Silly? Maybe. However, it is a strange little thing; after a while, you *really* want to draw another smiley face, write another *"YAY,"* or stick another sticker on the page. These small triumphs get momentum moving in your favor and get you in the mindset that this is working and you're doing pretty well.

Do I deserve a check mark today? What happens if you absentmindedly pop a sugary mint in your mouth or consciously give in to a craving? Do you have to start over at Day 1? Would a check mark be cheating?

Keep in mind that perfection is the goal but rarely the reality. Freeing your body and brain from the stronghold of sugar is a big thing, and no one moves through their sugar-free month without a few weak moments.

When filling out your report card, practice self-compassion rather than self-criticism. If you slip up, whether intentionally or unintentionally, get right back on track. Don't let defeating thoughts sneak in, e.g. *I already blew it today. I might as well give up and start over tomorrow.*

If you return to the no-sugar ground rules (pg. 15) for the rest of the day, you learned a lot and deserve that check mark. If your slip feels more like a free fall, leave that day unchecked and remind yourself that the slip-up doesn't mean you are a failure; it means you are human. At the end of the month, you can elect to add additional days to make up for the unchecked days or put a smile on your face and feel good about how many days you succeeded.

ZERO SUGAR / ONE MONTH
GROUND RULES

PRIMARY GOAL: Eliminate added sugar from your diet for 30 consecutive days.

Rules for Avoiding Added Sugar

Avoid foods and drinks with sugar listed as one of the first three ingredients. If a packaged food or drink has sugar listed as one of the top three ingredients, don't eat it. Note that sugar goes by different names, including corn syrup, dextrose, maltodextrin, fruit juice concentrate, and sucrose. See a more complete list in the FAQ section (pg. 18).

When in doubt, do without. In other words, if you're not sure if a food contains added sugar, don't eat it.

Some natural sugar is allowed. Natural sugar locked inside whole foods, such as fruit, yogurt, nuts, and seeds, is allowed. However, isolated natural sweeteners, such as honey and dried fruits, should be avoided. See the FAQ section (pg. 18) for more on fruit and natural sweeteners.

Avoid fruit juice. 100% fruit juice is low in fiber and high in fructose. It absorbs into your system quickly and converts to fat easily. On top of that, some fruit juices contain added sugar. For these reasons, fruit juice should be avoided. *Exception: A tablespoon or two of lemon or lime juice squeezed into a drink or recipe as a flavor enhancer is acceptable.*

Noncaloric sugar substitutes can be used for the first few weeks. However, you'll be asked to stop using them for the final week. See the FAQ section (pg. 18) for details.

 Tip Jar

When you turn a packaged food over to read the ingredient list, remember that ingredients are listed by quantity. So the closer the ingredient is to the beginning of the list, the more the food contains.

Rules for Eating

Eat whole foods. Eat unprocessed foods, such as meat, fish, eggs, unsweetened dairy products (cheese, cream, yogurt, etc.), vegetables, low-sugar fruits (berries, melons, etc.), raw nuts and seeds, extra-virgin oils, herbs, and spices. If you prefer a plant-based diet, low-processed grains (quinoa, steel-cut oats, wild rice, etc.) and soy-based proteins (tofu, tempeh, etc.) can be eaten.

 Tip Jar

Packaged nuts and seeds are often roasted in cheap, unhealthy oils and then flavored. For smooth sailing during your sugar-free month, choose raw nuts and seeds. Toasting enhances the flavor and crunch, so feel free to pop them in a 350°F (180°C) oven for 5 to 8 minutes or until fragrant and golden.

Eat a lower-carb/better-carb diet. By cutting out foods with sugar listed as one of the top three ingredients, you eliminate most nutrient-poor, high-carb foods. Avoiding these foods stabilizes your blood sugar, helping you control hunger and cravings naturally. To accelerate your transition to a sugar-free lifestyle, I recommend limiting flour and starch and boosting your intake of healthy fats to at least 50% of your daily calories. Foods that contain flour and starch include breads, cereals, grains, rice, potatoes, and corn. Healthy fats can be found in animal and plant-based foods. Recommended food lists are provided on page 22.

Don't get too hungry. It's tempting to undereat or significantly reduce your calorie intake during *Zero Sugar / One Month*. However, this isn't a diet with a specific calorie target. It's a program to build a sugar-free foundation. Your body will need some assistance as it transitions away from sugar, so eat when you're hungry. You'll find that hunger naturally diminishes within 7 to 10 days, leaving you feeling comfortable and in control of how much you eat.

Be cautious of packaged snacks. While they hold the promise of being healthy, many convenient snacks, such as granola, energy bars, trail mix, and mass-produced keto snacks, are refined, sweetened, and filled with dodgy ingredients, making them no better than the junk food they're replacing.

Avoid sweetened homemade snacks. Yes, there are "healthy" snack recipes with ingredients that technically fit our ground rules. However, they're easy to overeat and calorie-dense—two factors that can derail progress. At the end of the day, a cookie is still a cookie, even if it is made with dates, almond flour, or monk fruit.

Drink unsweetened drinks. Beverages sweetened with nonnutritive sweeteners, such as diet sodas and artificially flavored sports drinks, aren't recommended but can be used as a crutch at the start of the challenge. You'll be asked to wean yourself off all sweetened drinks by the final week. Approved drinks include plain water, carbonated water (sparkling or mineral water, seltzer), coffee, and hot or iced tea. Heavy cream or half-and-half can be added to coffee or tea.

FAQS

Here's the fine print to clear up some frequently asked questions.

Q: What should my macros be? *Zero Sugar / One Month* is focused on eliminating added sugar from your diet. Therefore, a specific macronutrient breakdown (percentage of carbs, fat, and protein) hasn't been set. With that said, you'll find that cravings and hunger are diminished by eating a lower-carb/better-carb diet. Everyone's carbohydrate tolerance is different. However, as a general guideline, aim to consume no more than 125 grams of carbohydrates per day. If you prefer to follow a keto diet, consume fewer than 50 grams daily. (Note: When I refer to grams of carbs, I'm referring to total carbs, not net carbs.)

Q: Can I eat fruit?

A: Fruit doesn't contain added sugar, but most fruits are sweet. There are no limitations placed on whole fruit at the beginning of the program. However, as you progress, you'll be encouraged to reduce your fruit intake to no more than two servings per day, reducing your dependence on the sweet taste.

Q: Can I have honey, agave nectar, maple syrup, molasses, or dates (dried fruit)?

A: These sweeteners come from natural sources, but they get much of their sweetness from fructose, which is a type of sugar that's easily metabolized into fat by your liver. Because of that fact and the intense sweetness of these products, you're encouraged to avoid them during *Zero Sugar / One Month.*

Q: To be "sugar-free," must I avoid natural sugar or trace amounts of sugar?

A: Many foods contain natural sugar or trace amounts of added sugar. Naturally occurring sugars found in unsweetened dairy products, fruit, and other whole foods can be included in your diet. If a packaged food contains added sugar but the added sugar isn't one of the top three ingredients, the food contains trace amounts of sugar and can be consumed during the challenge.

Q: What are common names for sugar?

A: Sugar has many aliases. Avoid these common names for added sugar: corn syrup, dextrose, fructose, fruit juice concentrate, glucose, high-fructose corn syrup, lactose, maltodextrin, maltose, and sucrose. Additional less common but equally sneaky names for sugar: agave nectar/syrup, barley malt, blackstrap molasses, brown rice syrup, coconut sugar, date sugar, evaporated cane juice, galactose, dextrin, malt syrup, turbinado sugar.

Q: Can I use sugar substitutes?

A: Artificial sweeteners (Splenda, Equal, Sweet'N Low) and sweeteners derived from natural sources (stevia, monk fruit) can be used at the onset of the program. However, you'll be prompted to stop using them for the final week.

Sweetness without nutritional value offers partial but not complete activation of the food reward pathways. In the moment, you'll enjoy eating or drinking the treat. However, by consuming it, you've kept your desire for sweet foods alive, making it hard to live comfortably without sugar. Bottom line: Swapping regular snacks and desserts for sugar-free versions does nothing more than kick your sugar habit down the road, leaving the door to temptations and cravings wide open.

Q: What are common names of nonnutritive sugar substitutes?

A: Common names include allulose, acesulfame-K, aspartame (Equal), erythritol, maltitol, monk fruit, saccharin (Sweet'N Low), sorbitol, stevia, sucralose (Splenda), and xylitol.

Q: Can I eat dark chocolate?

A: I recommend avoiding dark chocolate during *Zero Sugar / One Month*. It's possible to find dark chocolate made with noncaloric sweeteners or little added sugar, making it a snack that technically abides by the ground rules. However, this is a processed food that will keep your desire for sweets alive. Make a clean break from all types of chocolate and you'll wonder what all the fuss was about 30 days from now.

Q: Can I drink diet soda and similar beverages?

A: These noncaloric drinks are often sweetened with artificial sweeteners. You can consume them at the start of the challenge but will be asked to remove them from your diet for the final week.

Q: Can I drink alcohol?

A: Ideally, alcohol is avoided during *Zero Sugar / One Month*. However, the consumption of lower-carb alcoholic beverages, such as low-carb beer, dry wine, and pure spirits (vodka, gin, tequila, rum, and whiskey), isn't forbidden. I'll attach a warning label: drinking alcohol lowers inhibitions, making it hard to resist the tempting call of sugar and refined foods. Proceed at your own risk.

Q: What if I "slip" or fall off the wagon?

A: To err is human; to recover immediately, divine. *Zero Sugar / One Month* challenges you to avoid added sugar for 30 days. However, as a human, it's not out of the realm of possibility that you might subconsciously pop a sweet something into your mouth or give in to temptation during a moment of weakness. If that happens, get back on track immediately. No more sugar. If the slip triggered hunger, eat something from the approved food list (pg. 22) and move on.

Q: Can I snack?

A: You can snack between meals if you so desire. However, I recommend choosing low-carb/high-fat snacks, such as cheese, hard-boiled eggs, a beef stick, raw nuts and seeds, or veggies and dip, to avoid stimulating your sweet tooth.

Q: Can I practice intermittent fasting during the program?

A: Yes. If you're comfortable with intermittent fasting, you can continue to practice it during *Zero Sugar / One Month*.

DAY O PREP

It's time to prep for success! We'll refer to this section as Day 0 Prep because the tasks are intended to be completed prior to your start date. I realize that you may not be able to review all of the resources in one day. Therefore, if you need a few Day 0s, take them! But not too many. Your first task is to pick your start date.

PICK YOUR START DATE

The date you choose as your official Day 1 is up to you. However, I encourage you to begin within five days of acquiring this program. That will give you sufficient time to prep for the challenge without a dip in motivation.

I will start my 30-day sugar-free period on _____.

ZERO SUGAR
FIRST-TIER FOOD LIST

or What to Eat When Sugar is off the Table

The following lists include whole foods that are naturally low in sugar and carbohydrates. Use these foods as a foundation for meals and snacks during *Zero Sugar / One Month*.

MEAT & EGGS

- Beef
- Bison
- Chicken
- Duck
- Eggs
- Lamb
- Organ meats
- Pork
- Turkey
- Veal
- Venison

FISH & SEAFOOD

- Catfish
- Crab
- Crawfish
- Flounder
- Haddock
- Herring
- Lobster
- Mackerel
- Mussels
- Oysters
- Salmon
- Sardines
- Scallops
- Shrimp
- Squid
- Tilapia
- Trout
- Tuna

NON-STARCHY VEGETABLES

- Artichoke
- Asparagus
- Bamboo shoots
- Bean sprouts
- Bok choy
- Broccoli
- Brussels sprouts
- Cabbage
- Cauliflower
- Celery
- Collard greens
- Cucumbers
- Eggplant
- Garlic
- Green beans
- Jicama
- Kale
- Kohlrabi
- Leafy greens
- Leeks
- Mushrooms
- Mustard greens
- Okra
- Onions
- Peppers
- Radishes
- Snow peas
- Spinach
- Summer squash
- Swiss chard
- Tomatoes
- Zucchini

NUTS & SEEDS

- Almonds
- Brazil nuts
- Cashews
- Chia seeds
- Flaxseeds
- Hazelnuts (filberts)
- Hemp seeds
- Macadamia nuts
- Pecans
- Pine nuts
- Pistachios
- Pumpkin seeds
- Sesame seeds
- Sunflower seeds
- Walnuts

FRUITS

LOW-SUGAR FRUITS

- Avocados
- Blackberries
- Lemons
- Limes
- Olives
- Raspberries
- Strawberries

MODERATE-SUGAR FRUITS

- Apples
- Apricots
- Blueberries
- Cantaloupe
- Grapefruit
- Honeydew melon
- Kiwi
- Oranges
- Peaches
- Pomegranate
- Plums
- Watermelon

DAIRY

- Cheese
- Cottage cheese
- Half-and-half
- Heavy cream
- Unsweetened Yogurt

FATS & OILS

- Avocado oil
- Butter
- Cocoa butter
- Coconut oil
- Flaxseed oil
- Ghee
- Lard
- MCT oil
- Olive oil
- Palm oil
- Tallow
- Walnut oil

MISCELLANEOUS

- Apple cider vinegar and other vinegars
- Bone broth
- Coconut cream
- Full-fat veggie dip and salad dressing
- Herbs and spices
- Kimchi
- Mustard
- Sour cream
- Tofu
- Unsweetened dairy-free milk (e.g., almond milk, coconut milk, hemp milk)

ZERO SUGAR
SECOND-TIER FOOD LIST

The following foods can be consumed to round out an enjoyable diet, but due to being processed or having too much starch or natural sugar, it is best to limit your intake.

PROCESSED MEATS

- Bacon
- Beef jerky
- Deli meats
- Pork rinds (cracklings)

STARCHY VEGETABLES

- Acorn squash
- Butternut squash
- Carrots
- Corn
- Garden (English) peas
- Parsnips
- Potatoes (sweet, russet, white)
- Pumpkin
- Rutabaga (Swede)
- Taro
- Turnips
- Water chestnuts
- Yams

HIGH-SUGAR FRUITS

- Banana
- Cherries
- Grapes
- Mango
- Pear
- Pineapple

NUT & SEED BUTTERS

- Almond butter
- Cashew butter
- Sunflower butter
- Macadamia butter
- Natural peanut butter

LEGUMES (BEANS)

- Black beans
- Black-eyed peas
- Chickpeas/ garbanzo beans
- Edamame
- Great northern beans
- Kidney beans
- Lentils
- Lima beans
- Navy beans
- Peanuts
- Pinto beans

GRAINS

- Barley
- Oats
- Popcorn
- Quinoa
- Rice (brown or wild)

MISCELLANEOUS

- Condiments (e.g., cream cheese, mayonnaise, no-sugar-added sauces, and ketchup)
- Fermented drinks (e.g., kombucha, kefir)
- Tempeh
- Seitan
- Unsweetened protein powder

SNEAKY SUGAR

Sugar is added to many common and seemingly healthy foods. Here's a list of surprising foods that often contain sugar within the top three ingredients.

- Bacon
- Barbecue sauce
- Beef jerky
- Beef sticks
- Bread
- Breakfast cereal
- Canned baked Beans
- Canned fruit
- Cereal bars
- Coffee drinks
- Dark chocolate
- Dairy-free milk
- Energy bars
- Fruit juice
- Granola
- Ice cream
- Iced tea
- Instant oatmeal
- Ketchup
- Low-fat Yogurt
- Miracle whip
- Pasta sauce
- Peanut butter
- Protein bars
- Relish
- Salad dressings
- Sports drinks
- Trail mix

Remember that sugar goes by many different names. Some foods on this list do not have "sugar" on the ingredient list. Instead, they contain a sugar alias. Corn syrup, dextrose, maltodextrin, fruit juice concentrate, and sucrose are common alternate names, but there are many more! See a full list in the FAQ section (pg. 18).

Tip Jar: Getting Back in Touch with True Hunger

Modern-day convenience meals and snacks contain a magical combination of sugar, fat, and salt that keeps you coming back for more. These processed and refined foods have been engineered to increase appetite, making it hard to tell the difference between needing nourishment (aka true hunger) and a manufactured drive to eat (aka false hunger).

Zero Sugar / One Month cuts out sugar, bringing you back in touch with true hunger. Understanding how much food it takes to leave you feeling satisfied helps fine-tune your healthy diet. Here are some easy methods for estimating your food intake.

 Use the palm of your hand to estimate a portion of meat, fish, or poultry.

 Use your fist to estimate a portion of fruit or starchy vegetables (raw).

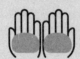 Two cupped hands are used to estimate a portion of non-starchy vegetables (raw).

 Your thumb is equal to a portion of hard cheese, seeds, or nut butter.

 One cupped hand represents a portion of nuts, beans, or grains.

 Use the tip of your thumb to estimate a portion of butter, oil, or other fats.

SET UP TEMPTATION-FREE ZONES

With your start date in mind, it's time to temptation-proof your home, office, and any other living area where sweet temptations reside.

10 Steps to Temptation-Free Zones

1. **Out of sight, out of mind.** Remove any processed food or refined carb snacks from your kitchen counters (cookies, cake, candy, chips, crackers, white bread, buns, etc.).

2. **Freshen up your kitchen.** Fill your eating areas with reminders of healthy living. Place low-sugar fruits, like avocados, lemons, and limes, in a decorative bowl. Display cut flowers alongside a pitcher of filtered water with lemon slices. Open the window blinds to bring in the sun.

3. **Have contingency eating plans.** Hunger and social events can be unpredictable. Having acceptable foods on hand will keep you on track. Pack and carry emergency items that hold up well without refrigeration, such as raw almonds in a baggie, beef sticks, or a packet of unsweetened almond butter.

4. **Be "no, thank you" ready.** Friends and family will offer sweet treats. A straightforward "no, thanks" and a change of subject may do the trick. For those who want to love you with food, artfully say no by making a non-food request. "No, thank you. But I would love a glass of water."

5. **Clean out snack food drawers.** Replace sugary snacks with raw nuts and seeds or non-food items (measuring cups, recipes, etc.). If family members are unwilling to live without processed snacks in the house, move them to your pantry and place in a container with a lid.

6. **Clean out your cereal/cracker/chip storage area.** Replace the refined-carb items with low-carb snacks like unsweetened beef sticks or beef jerky, dry storage vegetables (e.g., sweet potatoes, onions, garlic), healthy oils (e.g., coconut, olive, avocado oils), carbonated waters, tea or coffee supplies, etc.

7. **Set up your refrigerator for success.** Place salad ingredients in an easy-to-grab area and have a jug of unsweetened iced tea handy. Keep ready-to-eat raw vegetables with full-fat dip on a convenient shelf alongside hunger-satisfying snacks, like hard-boiled eggs and pre-sliced cheese. Hide your housemate's tempting snacks or drinks in drawers or low shelves.

8. **Rearrange your freezer.** Pack it with bags of frozen vegetables (e.g., broccoli, cauliflower, snap peas, soup vegetables, green beans) and bags of frozen berries (e.g., blueberries, raspberries, strawberries). Hide less-healthy foods that your family might want on hand (e.g., ice cream, frozen pizza, snack foods) in the back where they are inconvenient to grab.

9. **Rearrange your pantry.** Stock your pantry shelves as if they are shelves at the grocery store. You want the "best" (i.e., healthiest) foods at eye level and the "worst" foods placed up high or down low. For example, put low-sugar cooking ingredients, salad dressings, and spices at eye level. Move packaged snacks, noodles, grains, and baking items to the top and bottom shelves.

10. **Remove all "secret stashes."** Go through your home, office, or car and remove any processed snacks or sugary treats from the bedroom nightstand, living room end table, desk drawers, glove compartment, purse, etc.

Tip Jar

Low-fat dairy foods often contain added sugar. Stick with the original full-fat varieties of dips, dressings, and yogurts (4–5% milk fat) during your sugar-free month for more hunger control.

DAY 0 SELF-ASSESSMENT

Take this self-evaluation the day before starting *Zero Sugar / One Month* or the morning of Day 1 to capture your baseline data. You will be reminded to retake the assessment on Day 10, Day 20, and Day 30.

Body Stats

Below you'll find room to record your current body measurements. If you do not have access to all of the measurements, simply record what you can.

Current Weight _____

Body Fat % _____

BMI _____

Fasting Blood Sugar _____

Gathering Stats

Body Fat %—Some bathroom scales measure body fat percentage. If your scale does not have this feature, ask your doctor or a local gym if they have a body composition scale.

BMI—Body mass index (BMI) is a measure of body fat based on height and weight. You can google "BMI calculator" to find your result online.

Fasting Blood Sugar—Fasting blood sugar is a measure of your morning blood sugar level after an overnight fast. Less than 100 mg/dL (5.6 mmol/L) is normal.

Measurements

Measure against bare skin. Use a flexible tape measure or a string that you can later hold up to a ruler to determine your measurements.

Chest (measure around the
fullest area)
_____

Waist (measure one inch
(2.5cm) above your belly
button)
_____

Hips (measure around the
fullest area with your heels
together)
_____

Right Arm (measure around
the fullest area above the
elbow)
_____

Right Thigh (measure around
the fullest area)
_____

Photos

You may be tempted to skip the photos. But if you do, you will be kicking yourself at the end of your journey! You can take selfies or ask a friend for help. I recommend taking a full-body picture from the front, back, and side, and a close-up of your face. You'll be happiest with your comparison if you wear the same clothing in each photo session and stand in front of the same solid background.

Progress Chart

With the *Zero Sugar / One Month* program, success is measured in more ways than the scale. By comparing your Progress Chart answers today with your answers throughout the 30-day period, you'll clearly see that life is better on the other side of sugar!

NON-SCALE ASSESSMENT	TRUE	MOSTLY TRUE	(UNSURE) NEUTRAL	MOSTLY UNTRUE	NOT TRUE
My pants fit loose.					
My rings fit loose.					
My sleep is restful.					
My ability to focus is strong.					
My energy level is high.					
My sugar cravings are low.					
My joints are pain-free.					
My ability to cope with stress is high.					
My outlook is positive.					
My nose is rarely stuffy.					
I do not snore at night.					
My skin is clear of blemishes.					
There is no swelling in my legs.					
My sense of accomplishment is high.					

ZERO SUGAR / ONE MONTH
TIMELINE
A day-by-day account of what you might be feeling and experiencing during your month without sugar

Days 1–3 You're experiencing everything: excitement, fear, confidence, panic, and a few odd belly gurgles. You are doing okay, but your body and brain are feeling blindsided and nagging at you to go back to your old habits by turning on cravings, creating brain fog, fatigue, and grumpiness. The big question in your head is, *"Did I make the right choice?"* Of course, you did! It is normal to feel like you're riding an emotional and physical roller coaster at the start. Stick with it. It gets easier. You are right where you need to be.

Days 4–6 The fog is starting to lift, and you have a general sense of feeling better, but you're frustrated because you are <u>fill in the blank</u> (i.e., hungry, hangry, anxious, cranky, irritable). What you can't see is that your body is already adapting. Without added sugar and refined carbs, your blood sugar level has stabilized, bringing physical cravings under control (emotional cravings are still there), and your body is learning to use fat for fuel. The transition from being a sugar-burner to a fat-burner is not yet complete, but the resulting high energy and accelerated fat loss is right around the corner.

Days 7–10 The transition period is wrapping up, and you can feel it. You note times of high energy and clarity. The ill feelings are not entirely gone but have diminished as the enzymes and pathways needed for efficient fat breakdown increase. Your body is becoming more metabolically flexible, meaning it can switch between running on free fatty acids (fat) or glucose (sugar) with ease. Now is a great time for some self-care. Resist the urge to push your body by undereating. This reactive strategy can backfire, leading to cravings and fatigue. Also, don't feel bad about going to bed early for the next few days. It's a great way to give your body (and mind) some well-deserved rest as it works extra hard to become a better fat burner.

Day 11: You're feeling okay physically, but the newness has worn off, and the light at the end of the 30-day tunnel is still dim. These middle-of-your-goal blahs are expected and uncomfortable, but hang in there because true change is happening inside of you. You are right on track.

Days 12–14 Your body has adapted to running on fat for energy, reducing hunger and making it easier to extend the period between meals and say "no, thank you" to temptations. As a result, you notice that your pants are looser, your mind is clearer, and your sleep is more restful. However, environmental cues and emotional ties to sugary treats linger, creating Automatic Negative Thoughts (aka ANTs) that make you question whether this no-sugar thing is really worth it. It is! You've already conquered one-third of the challenge and are speeding toward the midway point; don't you want to stick it out to see what happens?

Day 15 It's hump day! You have made it to the halfway point of your 30-day journey! That deserves a big pat on the back! You still experience the blahs, but these periods have shortened to the point where you see how you truly are okay without sugar. You've come this far, don't stop before the magic happens!

Days 16–20 The changes are undeniable. You no longer keep the dog awake with your snoring. There is no longer a need for an afternoon nap, and your taste buds have recovered from the intensely sweet assault of processed snacks, opening up a whole new foodie world where the pleasant taste of subtly sweet foods like berries, nuts, and even veggies shine through. These "aha" moments pique your interest, making you wonder what else you've been missing all these years.

Day 21 You wake up this morning knowing that 20 no-sugar days are in the books! Yay! The periods of happiness, confidence, and high energy are lasting longer than before. However, life stressors still push your buttons, causing that little voice inside to question the harm of *"one little bite"* and sparking fears that you're not as far along mentally or physically as you should be. It is common to experience boredom and burnout at this point. Remind yourself that the hard days are the best days because when you make it through them, real progress happens.

Days 22–23 These couple of days will be mixed with feelings of *"I've got this in the bag"* to *"Aren't we there yet?"* This mental ping-pong match can lead to some unusual experiences. Have you dreamt about sugar yet? Food dreams can leave you scratching your head but know that it is normal for thoughts of sugar to pop into your head overnight or during a daydream. It is tempting at this stage to just push your body over the finish line. Remind yourself that you get what you want when you give your body what it needs. Restock your "Survival Pack (Day 4)," eat real food when you're hungry, and enjoy your day!

Day 24 You have officially entered your final week! Wow! You've rounded the corner, and you're headed for home. The cheerleader in your head is chanting *rah, rah, rah!* It is time to up your game and cross the finish line in style. This final week, you'll cut out non-caloric sweeteners and reduce your fruit intake.

Days 25–27 You are breaking down barriers that have been in place for a long time, and it feels good—*Aah*. Sit in the peace of this moment and enjoy but stick with your one-day-at-a-time commitment. The finish line is in sight, but you still have to get to it. Speaking of that finish line. You've been thinking about it. Right? You may even be making plans for Day 31. That is a fun day to daydream about, yet it can also feel intimidating (even scary) to think about navigating life without the strangely comforting no-sugar boundary. No worries. The remaining daily guides will help you traverse this uncharted territory.

Days 28–29 You're *sooooo* close. Excitement is rising, and you feel so good about what you've accomplished that you begin to think 28 or 29 days is close enough. Nope. While you can count the remaining time in hours, quitting now has consequences, not the least of which is regret. Do you want to remember that you kind of completed a month without sugar or that you did it? Hint: There is nothing better than being able to say, *"I did it!"*

Day 30 Today, you complete your 30-day commitment! The journey was not perfect; no journey worth taking is. However, you stuck with it, proving that you can take on a challenge and not falter, give in, or make excuses. That is a *really* good feeling.

Day 31 You are officially a *Zero Sugar / One Month* alumni! Bask in the knowledge that you accomplished something that others just talk about doing. Well done!

DAILY FOCUS – AT A GLANCE

Each day of your *Zero Sugar / One Month* journey starts with a Daily Focus. The handy guide below shares all of them at-a-glance. You can use this collection to chart your progress and remember your daily intention.

Day 1: Take Action We live in the information age, so we have every opportunity to study and learn, but the only true teacher is action. Today, you're taking action! Give yourself a high-five!

Day 2: Be Prepared Sometimes, it feels like we live in a sugar-coated world. You can't control the world, but you can set up your living spaces so tempting treats are out of sight and out of mind.

Day 3: None Is Easier Than Some The easiest way to stay sugar-free is to eat *none* because *some* stimulates your appetite. Today, you're making your life easier by reminding yourself that "None is easier than some."

Day 4: Avoid Getting Too Hungry [Survival Pack] Give your body what it needs today and it will give you what you want tomorrow. Today, you're putting together a hunger survival pack and giving yourself permission to eat when you are hungry.

Day 5: Find Your Big WHY Pursuing a goal is enjoyable when you understand *why* you are taking action. Today, you are uncovering your "Big WHY" for going sugar-free, and it feels good!

Day 6: Get Your Emotions Working for You True motivation is not an external thing or event; it comes from within. Today, you are getting your emotions working for you to experience the truth that *life is SO much better on the other side of sugar!*

Day 7: Line Up Your Stoppers Today, you are disarming habitual sugar cravings by using Stoppers to stop overeating before it starts.

Day 8: Disrupt Your Routine Eliminating sugar from your daily routine initially feels uncomfortable, but you will adapt. In fact, it's written in your DNA. Not only are humans habitual creatures, but we're also highly adaptable.

Day 9: Don't Beat Yourself Up What has your body done for you today? A lot! Today, you set your focus on appreciating all of the amazing things your body is willing to do for you.

Day 10: Take the Path Less Traveled—Your Own It's easy to follow the crowd. But where is the crowd leading you? Today, you recommit to taking another step on your straight and narrow path to exceptional health.

Day 11: Make the Choice Avoiding sugar is a choice. Making that choice feels uncomfortable, but it unlocks a world of opportunities.

Day 12: Exterminating ANTs One thing can always be said about sugar. You never wake up wishing you had eaten more of it the night before. Today, you are making the conscious decision to stop overthinking and just do it!

Day 13: That Went Well There is more than one way to look at any situation, and you get to choose your focus. Today, you are directing your focus toward the good of life by acknowledging what went well.

Day 14: Feed True Hunger, Ignore False Hunger True hunger is driven by your body's physiological need for fuel, whereas false hunger is driven by other factors, such as habits, routines, whims, and scarcity. Today's hunger scale exercise gives you the tool to tell the difference.

Day 15: Don't Stop Before the Magic Happens! You are halfway there! Hooray! Don't stop before the magic happens!

Day 16: The Elimination Trifecta Today, you are taking the opportunity to up your game by avoiding the Elimination Trifecta—sugar, flour, and seed oils.

Day 17: Shift Your Perspective Situations are not under your control, but how you view them is. Today, you turn any frown upside down by choosing curiosity over self-judgment.

Day 18: Consistent Effort Matters You are still in the game, proving that you've got what it takes to see this challenge through. Today, you acknowledge the new, enjoyable healthy habits you've developed.

Day 19: One Day at a Time Today, you build your awareness that the only way to win the race is to keep moving forward one step at a time.

Day 20: Maybe I'm Okay Your hard work is paying off! There is still work to be done, but for today, you are okay.

Day 21: Escaping the Sugar Comfort Zone Comfort zones keep you stuck. Today, you are questioning your sugar comfort zone to pursue what you really want.

Day 22: Lean into the Feel-Good Truth Just as a fire won't keep burning without more logs, enthusiasm won't stay alive without a positive focus. Today, you are stoking your inner fire by leaning into the feel-good truth.

Day 23: Living Above Sugar To live a sugar-free life, you must rise above sugar. The climb has challenges, but once you are perched on top, the problem is beneath you and manageable.

Day 24: Shed the Crutches Today, your sugar-free transition takes flight with the elimination of excess sweetness.

Day 25: New Ways to Make Food Choices When sugar no longer dulls your senses and hijacks your brain chemistry, you are free to enjoy new flavors and effortlessly make better food choices.

Day 26: Is That the Finish Line I See? Today, you are looking beyond the finish line, developing a "day-after" game plan.

Day 27: You are Becoming Sugar-Free One of the pleasant side effects of your consistent efforts is that sugar is no longer in control. You are becoming sugar-free, and it feels good!

Day 28: Completing the Journey You have come a long way, but 28 days are not the same as 30. Today, you choose to keep your eye on the prize, upholding your 30-day commitment.

Day 29: Sticking with Your Healthy Habits Your hard work over the past month has set you up for a lifetime of healthy habits that are easy to follow, enjoyable, and effective. That feels good!

Day 30: You've Arrived at Your Destination! There is no more worthy pursuit than the pursuit of health. You have given yourself a wonderful gift, and there is so much freedom ahead because of your actions.

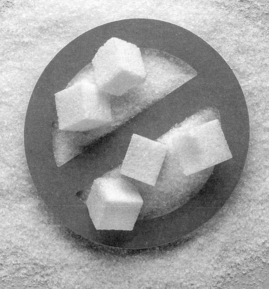

PART TWO

DAILY GUIDES

DAYS 1-10

A Sneak Peek at the Key Points Ahead

Day 1: Action is the best teacher.

Day 2: Out of sight, out of mind

Day 3: None is easier than some.

Day 4: Give your body what it needs and it will give you what you want.

Day 5: Find your "Big WHY" and motivation will follow.

Day 6: Life is so much better on the other side of sugar!

Day 7: Stoppers stop overeating before it starts.

Day 8: You're a habitual creature but also highly adaptable.

Day 9: Without question, your body is an engineering marvel.

Day 10: It's normal to experience uncomfortable feelings when working toward a goal.

DAY 1

TAKE ACTION

Daily Focus: We live in the information age, so we have every opportunity to study and learn, but the only true teacher is action. Today, you're taking action! Give yourself a high-five!·

Daily Motivation: *Setting Sail* Welcome to Day 1! Take a deep breath. Hold it for a few seconds. Breathe out. *(Whoooosh.)* If you're feeling a combination of excitement and nervousness, you're right where I expect to find you. It's normal to have mixed feelings when you set out to make a change. Your brain switches from *"Let's do this!"* to *"What are you doing?!?"* as if it's watching a ping-pong match. No worries. At the end of today, you get the satisfaction of checking the first box of your "I Did It!" report card. That reward will be yours because you did something most people aren't willing to do: You took action.

To settle first-day jitters and confirm why what you're doing is exactly what you're supposed to be doing, I want to share a short story about a teacher who gave three of his students an assignment. They were assigned to go out and learn as much as they could about how to sail a boat. Having no prior knowledge of sailing, the three students went their separate ways to complete their assignments.

The first student headed straight for the library, where he began a week of intense study. He learned everything he could about the different types of boats, the history of sailing, and the effects of the wind and seas on a sailing ship. By the end of the week, he felt confident he could answer any question his teacher might have about sailing a boat.

The second student decided he could learn through the experiences of others. Over the next week, he interviewed shipbuilders, sailors, and ship captains. He was given so many firsthand accounts about what to expect from the high seas that he felt he had already experienced it. He listened intently as the seafarers described in detail the mechanics of the boat and how to manage the sails. At the end of the week, he felt confident he could explain any aspect of sailing his teacher might ask of him.

The third student found a man who owned a sailboat and asked him for lessons. During the week that followed, the third student hoisted the sails, scrubbed the decks, navigated the waters, and piloted the boat during rough seas. He experienced excitement, boredom, exhaustion, and fear during his week, and he was humbled by the amount of knowledge and effort needed to sail a boat.

After one week, the class met again. The teacher took the three students down to a dock that moored three boats. The professor explained that their grade would be determined by how well each student could sail their boat.

The first two students climbed on board. They struggled to remember all they'd read and heard about sailing but soon realized that all their knowledge and enthusiasm provided no practical experience. Neither student could move the boat away from the dock. They failed the assignment.

The third student boarded his boat with trepidation, for this would be his first solo voyage. He remembered how he learned through his experiences to push the boat away from the dock. He recalled the precarious steering needed to properly position the vessel, and with strength and confidence, he raised the sails, catching the perfect wind.

The world we live in provides us with every opportunity to study and learn, but the only true teacher we can count on is action. Each day of your *Zero Sugar* journey comes with action steps that have been laid out in a logical sequence, building on each other in such a way that you'll grow more confident with each passing day. The first action step is agreeing to take action.

Daily Action: Commitment Over Convenience

Avoiding sugar for 30 days isn't convenient. It requires commitment. If you're merely interested in doing something, you do it only when it's convenient. When you're committed to doing something, you do it no matter what—even when it's inconvenient.

It's not convenient to pack your own healthy snacks or tell the waiter to hold the bread basket. But when you take side steps and give in to temptation, you'll be frustrated with your results and find yourself going around the same mountain month after month and year after year.

It's time to break that cycle—and this program is the tool you'll use to do so. Sign the Commitment Statement below and let's do this together!

Commitment Statement: I understand I'll have challenging days ahead. But I know that a new level of freedom, energy, and peace of mind is waiting for me on the other side of sugar. I accept this challenge and commit to applying the action steps laid out in the course for 30 days.

Signed _____

Daily Result and Reflections: Day 1 is in the books! You avoided foods and drinks with sugar listed as one of the top three ingredients. Flip back to page 13, fill in Day 1 of your "I Did It!" report card, and give yourself a well-deserved pat on the back.

Self-Reflection: Look back through your day and recall what kept you on track. Did you replay the "Setting Sail" story in your head? Did you have a strong desire to mark off Day 1 in your "I Did It!" report card? Was today's success chalked up to nothing more than sheer willpower? Don't judge your reason. Just write it down, along with any thoughts on what you could do better tomorrow.

What kept me on track today?

_____

_____

_____

_____

_____

_____

What could I do better tomorrow?

_____

_____

_____

_____

_____

DAY 2

BE PREPARED

Daily Focus: Sometimes, it feels like we live in a sugar-coated world. You can't control the world, but you can set up your living spaces so tempting treats are out of sight and out of mind.

Daily Motivation: *Stressed Out* It's 5:45 p.m. and you're finally home. What a day! You got a stain on your favorite shirt, your boss assigned another project on top of the three you still have on your desk, and that annoying coworker who never stops talking wouldn't stop talking. That was only Act One of this hectic day. Act Two began as you walked through the front door and heard "*What's for dinner?*"

You're stressed. You want comfort—and you want it now. Emotions take over and good judgment flies out the window. All you want to do is eat. How do you handle these out-of-control moments? Take a tip from the Boy Scouts and be prepared.

If you have the wrong foods in easy-to-grab places, you can subconsciously consume hundreds of empty calories before dinner gets on the table. On Day 0, you set up temptation-free zones (pg. 29) by removing sugary and refined carbs from your living spaces. (If you skipped that task, today would be a good day to complete it!) Those actions prepared you for the next time stress hits, which it will! Today, you'll dig a little deeper to determine if your home is working for or against your sugar-free goal.

Daily Action: Inventory Your Environment Scorecard

Place a check mark by each true statement:

KITCHEN COUNTERS

___ Counters are well organized, not cluttered.

___ The food preparation areas are brightly lit.

___ There are no breakfast cereals visible.

___ There are no breads or buns visible.

___ There are no refined snack foods visible (such as cookies, cakes, candies, crackers, chips).

___ There's at least one healthy food visible (such as an avocado, a tomato, an apple, or a lemon).

___ There's a pitcher of water or personal water bottle visible.

REFRIGERATOR

___ A favorite family photo or an inspirational item is near the door handle.

___ Precut or leftover non-starchy vegetables are stored inside.

___ Salad ingredients are in transparent containers or easy to see.

___ Any refined or high-carb snacks are hidden in the back or in a drawer. (Give yourself a check if there are no refined snacks.)

___ There are no sugary drinks in the refrigerator (such as soda, sports drinks, energy drinks, and sweetened tea.)

___ There are convenient fat or protein "emergency meals" available (such as hard-boiled eggs, cooked chicken or meat, smoked salmon, cooked shrimp, plain yogurt, and presliced cheese.)

FREEZER

___ There's at least one bag of frozen, non-starchy vegetables (such as broccoli, cauliflower, snap peas, or green beans.)

___ There's a bag of frozen berries.

___ There's no ice cream.

___ There are no high-carb convenience meals (frozen pizza, premade pasta meals, french fries, snack bites, etc.)

___ There's at least one no-sugar/low-carb convenient meal (cooked chicken, meat, or seafood, leftover entrée, etc.)

CUPBOARDS & PANTRY

___ There's no junk food drawer in the kitchen.

___ Raw nuts and seeds are found in a kitchen cupboard.

___ Spices are conveniently accessible in the kitchen (such as in a cupboard or on the countertop).

___ The pantry isn't located in the kitchen.

___ High-carb items (dry pasta, snack bars, crackers, prepackaged treats, etc.) are tucked away in a pantry away from the kitchen.

___ Healthy foods are in the front of the pantry shelving (such as canned vegetables, packaged salmon or tuna, nut butters, canned coconut milk, and olive or avocado oil.)

BONUS POINT

___ Give yourself a bonus point if there are no "secret stashes" of food outside the kitchen or pantry. (That is, there's no food in the bedroom, living room, home office, TV room, etc.)

_____

_____

SCORING BRACKETS

17–25 Doing Great! You've set up a temptation-free home!

12–16 Doing Okay. With a few more tweaks, your home will support your sugar-free lifestyle.

0–11 Your Environment Needs Work. No worries. Make changes based on what you learned and then retake the test.

Daily Result and Reflections: You did it! Flip to your "I Did It!" report card and give yourself a well-deserved check mark (or smiley face or sticker, or ... you get the idea)!

Self-Reflection: A temptation-free environment takes a few minutes to set up, but it protects you from the inevitable low-willpower moments of life. Think back over your day and identify one positive change you made that will make your journey easier.

A positive change I made today was:

_____

_____

_____

_____

_____

_____

DAY 3

NONE IS EASIER THAN SOME

Daily Focus: The easiest way to stay sugar-free is to eat *none* because *some* stimulates your appetite. Today, you're making your life easier by reminding yourself that "None is easier than some."

Daily Motivation: *Fearless Flight* One spring, a pair of birds built a nest in the vent above our guest bathroom. We heard them working hard to gather the twigs and scraps they needed to transform the small metal tube into a home. A few weeks later, we began to hear the soft, high-pitched chirps of their newly hatched family. It was fun to think about how the baby birds must be growing and to hear their cries increase in strength as they vied for the latest worm that their mom or dad brought back to the nest.

Then came the day for the young birds to leave the nest. The exit of the vent led out of the side of our house—about 10 feet off the ground— so the only way to leave was to fly. I imagine those fledglings must have hopped toward the edge with a great deal of trepidation. There would be no test flight. The moment their feet left the firm footing of their metallic home, their survival hinged on their ability to spread their wings and fly. It was literally a leap of faith. But I can also imagine how quickly fear was replaced with euphoria as they rose into the air and experienced the freedom of flight.

What does fear keep you from experiencing? Do you feel anxious about leaving the comfort of your current lifestyle? Do you fear how you'll feel without an afternoon sugar pick-me-up? Sometimes, we have to stop wondering what might happen and take a leap of faith.

The fledglings in our story could have stayed in the vent and eked out an okay life. But by choosing to take a big step, they got to experience the thrill of flight. Today's task will help you see that stepping out of your comfort zone—despite being scary—brings big rewards.

By taking the *Zero Sugar* challenge, you're taking a big step. Avoiding sugar like you're doing can be intimidating, which can lead to compromised thinking. For example, it's easy to tell yourself that "*A little bite won't hurt*" or "*If I eat this, it's not really cheating.*" Nope. We're not going to go there. Today's action step will cut off wayward thoughts before they can impact your actions. Today, you'll remind yourself that "None is easier than some."

The genius behind this simple phrase is that it protects you from your natural tendency as a human being. Humans have been hardwired from our primitive days to eat when food is available. So the mere act of eating—even a small bite of food—makes you want to keep eating.

When it comes to eating sugar, this drive to keep eating once you start is enhanced by emotional and physiological factors that make it even harder to control. Therefore, the easiest way to stay sugar-free is to eat *none* because *some* stimulates your appetite and triggers cravings.

Theresa embraced this mindset. In the past, she'd focus on how good a cookie or another treat would taste. Today, she thinks about how she'll feel if she eats it. Her "aha" moment came when she realized that the short-term pleasure that came from eating sweets led to longer-term regret.

Don't let compromised thinking convince you that a little taste of a sugary treat will satisfy your craving. It's a lie. The truth is that "None is easier than some." Take the leap of faith and completely break free from sugar. Yes, it's scary, but that fear is the only thing blocking your freedom.

Daily Action: None Is Easier Than Some.

To complete today's action step, write the phrase "None is easier than some" on a piece of paper or type a reminder into your phone. Put the paper somewhere where you'll encounter it multiple times today—maybe on your desk or in your front pants pocket. If you're using technology, set a reminder to ding every one to two hours for the remainder of the day. In other words, blaze the idea that "None is easier than some" into your brain.

Daily Result and Reflections: You did it! Cross off Day 3 on your "I Did It!" report card and congratulate yourself for not compromising.

Self-Reflection: The beauty of disrupting a compromising thought— "A small bite can't hurt"—with the beneficial thought—"None is easier than some"—is that it ends your brain's internal chatter. You don't have to fight with yourself over what to do. The decision has already been made. Those five words make life simpler and free up space in your mind that would otherwise be taken up by internal debate.

Think back to a time when you chose to avoid a sugary snack entirely. (Maybe it was today.) Now fast-forward to the present moment. Do you regret not eating that snack or are you proud of yourself for skipping it?

_____

_____

_____

_____

_____

_____

"Instead of forcing change, allow change to happen by giving your body what it needs to succeed."

AVOID GETTING TOO HUNGRY [SURVIVAL PACK]

Daily Focus: Give your body what it needs today and it will give you what you want tomorrow. Today, you are putting together a hunger survival pack and giving yourself permission to eat when you are hungry.

Daily Motivation: *Creatures of Habit* Ahh, the power of love. It can completely turn your world upside down and make you do some crazy things. I once went salmon fishing in the name of love. I was dating an avid outdoorsman and his family invited us to spend a weekend casting our rods and trying our luck during that year's great salmon run. We drove all night to a remote creek in rural New York. To save travel time, we ate meals from convenience stores and managed to grab two hours of sleep, sitting in the van before dawn broke. By sunrise, we'd gathered our gear and were hiking to "the spot," where we stood in icy cold water for the rest of the day. The only salmon I saw were two dead ones that floated by me as I stood in the chilly water, daydreaming about a flush toilet and calculating how many hours it would be until I could get a hot shower.

Nothing can make us step out of our normal routine like love. Nothing, that is, except the desire to take life by the reins and take back our health! Life has many priorities and it's common to let health goals drop down on our list. It's also common to experience the ignition of that internal spark that fires up our desire to change. The trigger for change can be anything from a health issue to a number we weren't expecting to see on the scale. Regardless of the stimulus, this is an empowering state to be in—one that comes with a sense we can achieve anything and everything! And we will! Change everything—all at once—today. This is where things get complicated.

First, we determine we're doing everything wrong. Next, we decide that we'll go against our basic instincts and natural tendencies and force change. We change the foods we eat, the times we eat, and the amount we eat. At the same time, we change how we move, going directly from couch potato to exercise guru, leaving our bodies to wonder if we've gone insane.

Committing to *Zero Sugar / One Month* is empowering and you might already be seeing positive changes in your body. This progress makes you want to see more—now! It seems logical that if this push is working, then a bigger push, such as cutting calories, eating only one meal a day, or adding intense exercise should get the job done faster. The reality is that if you push your body too hard, it will push back—and it has some powerful weapons, including cravings, hunger, and fatigue.

Instead of forcing change, allow change to happen by giving your body what it needs to succeed. Your goal for today (as with every day this month) is to avoid added sugar. If hunger arises, give yourself permission to eat. Don't focus on calories at this point. When your body has adapted to your new sugar-free diet, hunger will diminish naturally. In other words, give your body what it needs today and it will give you what you want tomorrow.

Daily Action: Create a Hunger Survival Pack

Today's action step is a fun one. Create a hunger survival pack, and when you're hungry, eat. Your survival pack will contain easy-to-grab foods that stop hunger in its tracks because they're low in carbs as well as high in fat and they contain protein. This combination stabilizes blood sugar, preventing blood sugar crashes that drive cravings.

To complete today's action step, gather convenient, hunger-satisfying foods. A list of ideas is provided below. You can put these items in a container or collect them on a shelf in your refrigerator. If you travel during the day, make a travel pack by placing shelf-stable foods, such as a packet of almond butter, raw almonds, and beef sticks, into a portable bag. Then, when hunger hits, eat.

- Deviled eggs
- Precooked meat
- Precooked chicken
- Precooked shrimp
- Presliced cheese
- Smoked salmon
- Veggies with full-fat dip or cream cheese
- Full-fat yogurt with fresh or frozen berries
- Full-fat cottage cheese with berries
- Stuffed olives
- Kimchi
- Single-serve packets of unsweetened almond butter
- Raw almonds or other nuts and seeds
- Beef sticks
- Beef jerky

RECIPE FOR SUCCESS

SURVIVAL PACK DEVILED EGGS

Deviled eggs are the perfect grab-and-go breakfast or afternoon snack. Having them on hand will help you stick with your no-sugar diet—even when life gets hectic.

SERVINGS 4 · SERVING SIZE: 3 DEVILED EGGS

6 hard-boiled eggs
2 tbsp full-fat mayonnaise
1 tbsp yellow mustard

2 tsp Dijon mustard
ground paprika, to taste

1. Cut the hard-boiled eggs in half lengthwise.

2. Place the yolks in a medium bowl and set the egg white halves aside. Smash the yolks with a fork.

3. Add the mayo and both mustards to the bowl. Mix well.

4. Spoon the mixture into the egg halves and sprinkle the paprika over the top.

Note: Miracle Whip is a popular substitute for mayonnaise. However, it contains high-fructose corn syrup, making it a poor choice. When choosing a commercial mayo, look for a brand made with avocado oil, such as Primal Kitchen.

NUTRITION PER SERVING		
Calories 171	Carbohydrates 1.3g	Sugars 0.9g
Fat 14.2g	Fiber 0.3g	Protein 9.7g

Daily Result and Reflections: You did it! Flip back to page 13, fill in the Day 4 box of your "I Did It!" report card, and give yourself a pat on the back.

Self-Reflection: If sugar and refined foods were a regular part of your diet before starting *Zero Sugar / One Month*, your body is currently going through a big change. It's feeling confused because the usual quick-energy carbs aren't coming in. Fortunately, your body will figure it out and switch to fat as its preferred fuel source, but that takes time. Today, you helped your body through this transition by feeding it. How did it feel to eat when you were hungry? Did you have trouble doing it? Were you left with a sense you were helping your body or betraying your goal? There's no right or wrong answer—just jot down your thoughts. Future you will appreciate them.

_____

_____

_____

_____

_____

_____

DAY 5

FIND YOUR BIG WHY

Daily Focus: Pursuing a goal is enjoyable when you understand *why* you are taking action. Today, you are uncovering your "Big WHY" for going sugar-free, and it feels good!

Daily Motivation: *Motivated by Vanity* I've found the secret to keeping my house clean: Invite people over. Whenever my house begins to win the war on clutter, I decide to have a dinner party. This provides me with the proper amount of disgust over the condition of my home. As the day my guests will arrive approaches, I get an incredible burst of cleaning energy. The filth doesn't stand a chance because I'm motivated by vanity!

I don't have qualms about revealing my dislike of cleaning. Fortunately, one of the few things I dislike more than cleaning is having people see how messy my house can get. I accept this as a kind of check and balance system for my life—and I've made it work.

We might find it hard to admit we can be motivated by vanity. I suppose it's because we don't want to appear shallow. But I suspect vanity plays a role in reaching many of our goals. For example, take weight loss. It's far nobler to eat right and exercise because you want to teach your children the joys of healthy living than to admit you want to be able to comfortably zip up your pants. As long as your approach is a healthy one, the motivating factor is inconsequential. If your doctor told you to cut out sugar to avoid diabetes, but you instead cut out sugar because you want to look good walking down the beach … well, you still improved your health.

Today, you'll do an exercise to uncover why avoiding sugar is important to you. This is a mental exercise and it's easy to brush these types of activities off as unimportant. But when you hit on the right reason or that compelling "why," you take action. Without it, you don't.

Daily Action: Finding Your "Big WHY"

For today's action step, you'll find your "Big WHY." In other words, what's your big reason (your "why") for wanting to stop eating sugar? To complete the exercise, you'll write down 15 things you love about your sugar-free life. Now, I get it. Today, life without sugar isn't a bed of roses. That's okay. You're invited to project into the future to complete your list.

Coming up with 15 things is important because you'll find that the first few you write down are the ones we all have in common. For example, "*I love being healthy*," "*I love the weight loss benefits*," and "*I love having energy*." Those are valid reasons and great quality of life factors. But despite being factual, they don't have that "it factor" that really *motivates* you.

I want you to come up with reasons that have meaning in your life. However, here's a list of examples to help get your creative juices flowing.

1. I love hearing my doctor say my blood work is perfect!

2. I love showing up at work/social events feeling confident and looking good.

3. I love being out with friends and not being focused on dessert and junk food.

4. I love that my kids aren't hooked on sugar.

5. I love having a clear mind and a stable mood.

6. I love having clear skin.

7. I love being able to fit comfortably in my clothes.

8. I love waking up in the morning without regrets about what I ate the night before.

9. I love that I'm living an authentic life and not sneak-eating.

10. I love bending and moving in my fit body.

11. I love finding new recipes that taste great without the "easy out" of sugar.

12. I love filling up on hearty, healthful food and not feeling bloated after a meal.

13. I love lying down at night, feeling accomplished for not taking the easy way out.

14. I love being able to exercise without joint pain.

15. I love not being gassy or having to worry about embarrassing digestive issues.

For this exercise, you have permission to be petty, vain, and self-serving. Try to do this exercise in one sitting and don't worry if you miss a comma here and there or if a few of your statements seem jumbled or redundant. The freedom to just blurt out thoughts on paper allows you to dig deep and find that hidden "why" that becomes your game-changer.

Now it's your turn! Take a deep breath, close your eyes, and put a smile on your face as you ask yourself (or your future self) what you love about being free from sugar. Start each statement with the words "I love." This helps you lean toward a positive outcome.

1. I love _____

2. _____

3. _____

4. _____

5. _____

6. _____

7. _____

8. _____

9. _____

10. _____

11. _____

12. _____

13. _____

14. _____

15. _____

Daily Result and Reflections: You did it! Give yourself another check mark! Wahoo!

Self-Reflection: Building a strong desire involves taking the time to understand what you truly want. This understanding allows you to pursue your goal with passion and enthusiasm. Take a moment to read your list. Allow yourself to feel any emotions that arise. Write down one reason that produced a good feeling or strong emotion. (Note: You might have many favorites, but this one reason is your "Big WHY" statement and can be used as your emotional trigger on Day 6.)

_____

_____

_____

_____

_____

_____

DAY 6

GET YOUR EMOTIONS WORKING FOR YOU

Daily Focus: True motivation is not an external thing or event; it comes from within. Today, you are getting your emotions working for you to experience the truth that *life is SO much better on the other side of sugar!*

Daily Motivation: *What's Your Motivation?* According to Jo Piazza, author of *Celebrity Inc.: How Famous People Make Money*, celebrity diet endorsers earn about $33,000 for each pound they lose. That's called *motivation!*

Believe me, if someone came to my door and offered me even half that amount, I'd put duct tape over my mouth and start doing jumping jacks before they left the house. Unfortunately, I don't foresee this offer in my or your near future. So we must look inside to find our own motivation. Fortunately, that's where true motivation resides.

Yes, outside influences can persuade us to act. However, *true* motivation isn't an external thing or event. You don't have to wait for a reward or some "thing" to happen to find it. Life doesn't need to become stress-free. You don't have to wait for that big project at work to be done and you don't need to have a $33,000 per pound contract waved in your face to experience motivation. All you need is to link emotion to your goal.

Emotion is the driving force that pushes you to achieve things. Think about it. Why did you learn how to drive a car? You have to admit that learning to drive is a bit scary. But you still wanted to learn because you equated driving to a feeling of freedom and independence. That emotional link helped you overcome fearful thoughts.

Making a declaration that you'll avoid sugar for 30 days is important. But adding emotions to that sugar-free goal provides the motivation needed to get the job done. This is where mantras fall short.

A mantra is a statement. A group of words stated without emotion means little. Try it for yourself. Using a mellow, conversational tone, state the phrase "Life is so much better on the other side of sugar." Feels rather bland, doesn't it? Now say the phrase again, but this time, put an emotional thrust behind it. When the words leave your lips, feel the energy build in your chest, spread to your back muscles, and expand within you. Ready? Say it with me: "Life is *so* much better on the other side of sugar!" Sit for a moment, feeling the expansiveness of that feeling burst inside you. That is what separates true motivation from mere words.

Now you might be thinking, that's a nice theory and might feel good at the moment, but I doubt it makes much difference over the long term. Well, I thought that too—until it led to one of the most mind-blowing moments of my life.

In January 2007, I vowed to run a marathon. I chose a race called the Flying Pig Marathon in Cincinnati, Ohio. (The name implies the thought that "I'll run a marathon when pigs fly.") When I started training, I not only got my body ready to run but also my mind. I did this by visualizing myself running across the finish line.

Every Saturday, I'd head out for my long training run. As the run finished, regardless of how I felt, I would run the last 100 feet like they were the final steps of my 26.2-mile journey. I'd get such a visual picture in my mind of that awesome moment that my arms would fly up in the air and tears would come to my eyes. I experienced the euphoria of crossing that finish line 17 times in my mind before the race even began.

I continued to link positive emotions to my desired outcome throughout the week. Day after day, I'd put myself in that same emotional state I felt at the end of my training runs and repeat this phrase: "*I'm absolutely certain in my ability to run the Flying Pig Marathon in 4:44*" (a time I had arbitrarily picked, but it just felt right). I enthusiastically repeated this phrase to myself three times a day every day and never let myself doubt I'd cross the finish line in 4 hours and 44 minutes, even on the days it didn't seem plausible because I was feeling worn out.

Race day finally came on Sunday, May 6. I'd completed a difficult physical training process that often required getting up before the sun on some very cold Saturday mornings, and while I was feeling some nervousness, I felt physically strong and I was glad the moment had arrived. I woke up that morning, said my phrase with emotion and confidence, and got ready to run.

The race was grueling. I endured warmer-than-expected temperatures, cramping in my legs, and a level of fatigue I'd never experienced before; but when the finish line came into view, I was overcome by emotion: My arms flew up in the air and my eyes filled with tears. I realized I was crossing the line at the exact time I had visualized: 4 hours and 44 minutes.

Daily Action: Adding Emotion to Your Goal

Yesterday (Day 5), you were asked to write down 15 reasons you love being sugar-free and pick out one that produced a particularly good feeling or strong emotion. That "Big WHY" statement will be your emotional trigger for today's action step.

To complete today's action step, you'll focus on your emotional trigger three times throughout the day (such as morning, afternoon, and evening). Consider setting a notification on your phone to act as a reminder. At each selected time, sit quietly with your eyes closed and recall your emotional trigger, such as *I love being able to fit comfortably in my clothes."* See an image of yourself living that reality. Feel the energy expand within your chest, spread to your back, and burst out of you. When you reach that state of positive energy, say to yourself: *"Life is SO much better on the other side of sugar!"*

I don't blame you if you initially feel silly doing this. But I promise you that if you do this three times today, you'll be amazed at how changed and motivated you feel. Pro tip: Make this a daily exercise and watch your motivation grow!

Daily Result and Reflections: You did it! This is starting to feel pretty good! Give yourself a check mark on your "I Did It!" report card.

Self-Reflection: Think back to a time in your life when you achieved something beyond your expectations. What was the emotional trigger that motivated you to accomplish that goal?

_____

_____

_____

_____

_____

_____

DAY 7

LINE UP YOUR STOPPERS

Daily Focus: Today, you are disarming habitual sugar cravings by using Stoppers to stop overeating before it starts.

Daily Motivation: *Hunger or Habit?* It's 8 p.m. and the TV is on, so bring on the snacks! Does this sound familiar? Are you really hungry for a snack or is this simply part of a habitual nightly ritual? Habits can get a solid grip on our lives. If we don't break them, they might break us.

Because eating habits are performed with little conscious thought, it's easy to stop paying attention to what you eat, how much you eat, where you eat, whether you're hungry, and the consequences of mindless snacking.

You can't break a habit if you don't see it. So the first step is to take a moment to think about your day. What are your habits pertaining to sugar and refined carbs? Do you always have a bedtime snack? Do you always have an energy drink in the afternoon? Is dessert a must after dinner? Do you need "just a little something sweet" after lunch? Whatever triggers your desire to consume sugar, you can disarm it with a simple tool called a Stopper.

A Stopper is an item, drink, or activity that allows you to separate from eating. Stoppers have immediate and long-term benefits. They immediately disrupt your desire to keep eating and, when used consistently, they break habit patterns.

The separation from eating that a Stopper creates is accomplished in different ways. For example, minty things, such as brushing your teeth or using mouthwash, freshen your mouth, making food less appealing. A Stopper that takes time to consume, such as a cup of hot tea after dinner, gives your stomach time to tell your brain that you're comfortably full.

Stoppers can even help you avoid snacking. Here's a trick to avoid late-night snacking that uses a packet of dental floss. Keep a floss dispenser in your living room. When you sit down at night to watch TV, floss. Once you've put forth the effort to clean your teeth, you'll be reluctant to dirty them again with more food. (And in 30 days, you'll have super-clean teeth. What a bonus!)

Consistent use of a Stopper can help you break habitual patterns that make sugar seem irresistible. There's a philosophy that states that habits aren't broken—they're just replaced by other habits. Let's say you identified your trouble time as being when the kids get home from school. Right before you expect them to walk through the door, brush your teeth. Do this consistently and you'll be surprised how soon your brain shifts from "It's time for a snack" to "It's time to brush my teeth."

For today's action step, you'll select a few Stoppers and make sure they're available at a moment's notice. I've provided a list of Stoppers below.

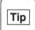 **Tip Jar**

To strengthen your brain's understanding that this item or activity means eating has ended, pick something that's only used as a Stopper. For example, set aside a special flavor of sugar-free gum or tea you only consume after a meal or make dental floss your go-to Stopper when watching TV. The quicker your brain gets the message that eating has ended, the easier it will be for you to avoid sugar.

Daily Action: Line Up Your Stopper(s)

When choosing a Stopper, feel free to be creative. Select something that takes a long time to consume, changes the taste in your mouth, or signals that eating has come to an end in a symbolic way. For example, right after a meal, slowly sip a cup of hot tea, pop a piece of minty sugar-free gum into your mouth, or fold a napkin over your plate. You'll find you naturally move away from the urge to keep eating.

Here's a list of Stoppers to choose from. Circle the ones that will work for you or use the blank space to write in a unique Stopper:

- Chew a piece of sugar-free gum.
- Stick a flavored toothpick in your mouth.
- Drink hot or cold tea. (Minty or other strong flavors work well.)
- Take a supplement best taken on an empty stomach (which works well for avoiding snacking).
- Sip a salty electrolyte drink.
- Sip bubbly water (such as seltzer or mineral water).
- Eat one Brazil nut. (It's big and rich in healthy fats, selenium, and magnesium.)
- Place a napkin over your plate.
- Turn off the kitchen light after dinner.
- Walk your dog.
- Floss your teeth.
- Brush your teeth.
- Use teeth whitening strips.
- Swish your mouth with mouthwash.
- Move to the living room and do a crossword puzzle.
- Paint your fingernails.
- Play the guitar, piano, or another instrument.
- _____

Daily Result and Reflections: You did it! One week is in the bag! Go get that "I Did It!" check mark recorded on your report card!

Self-Reflection: Stoppers are pattern disruptors. When you use one, you quiet the rebellious child inside that wants more and ease into acceptance that the meal is over. Write down a Stopper you used today and record your experience.

_____

_____

_____

_____

_____

_____

DAY 8

DISRUPT YOUR ROUTINE

Daily Focus: Eliminating sugar from your daily routine initially feels uncomfortable, but you will adapt. In fact, it's written in your DNA. Not only are humans habitual creatures, but we're also highly adaptable.

Daily Motivation: *The Alternate Route* I'm always amazed when I watch a squirrel walk across a power line. I was driving down a highly trafficked street when I last observed one of these fearless feats. I wondered why squirrels often choose this route to get to the other side of the road. To me, it seems they're tempting fate. One false step, and if the fall doesn't get them, the traffic surely will. But then I realized that squirrels must look at the problem of crossing a street differently than a person does.

The squirrel has two options: Run fast across the road and hope not to get squashed or navigate the high wire. The high wire must look like a perfectly sane solution to the squirrel because climbing trees and maneuvering over small branches is part of their daily lives. How ingenious! Instead of giving up and feeling hopeless about their ability to dodge all those cars, this common, ordinary backyard critter found an alternate route.

Finding a different path is challenging for humans because of our habitual nature. This isn't always a bad thing. Having routines makes life simple. However, routines can lead us down paths we don't want to go. This is often true with sugar. We fall into patterns, such as coffee needs two sugars or a sweet dessert is a must. When these things don't happen, we feel weird. Something's out of place. It's uncomfortable.

By following the *Zero Sugar / One Month* program, you're creating a new sugar-free habit. You're undoubtedly still experiencing uncomfortable periods when your body doesn't feel right without sugar. But stick with it and the magic will happen! David experienced this magic after decades of sugary indulgences. He grew up eating Fruit Loops and Frosted Flakes for breakfast and ate candy and drank Coke almost daily. For school lunch, his mom would pack a peanut butter/marshmallow/jelly sandwich, a Hostess cupcake, and a small bag of Fritos. As an adult, he switched to a no-sugar diet with great success, losing more than 50 pounds as well as his desire for sugar products. The transformation was so complete that he developed a distaste for sweets, finding it effortless to avoid them. He feels amazing, finds that his clothes fit better, and feels like he got his body back.

The reality is there are countless ways to go through your day. So you're free to change what's not working for you (such as eating sugar). Yes, it will feel awkward for a while, but you'll be amazed at how quickly your body and mind accept change. Want proof? For today's action step, we lighten things up a bit with a fun exercise to illustrate how today's uncomfortable change becomes tomorrow's comforting new habit.

Daily Action: Take an Alternate Route

Today's task asks you to change up a habitual pattern. You can choose anything you'd like, but make it small and easy to accomplish. Here are a few ideas:

- Change your seat at the dinner table or in the TV room.
- Sleep on the other side of the bed.
- Go in the reverse direction during your morning walk.
- Take a different route to work.
- Have a cup of tea instead of coffee.
- Use a different coffee mug.
- Use your standing desk at work.
- Start your work project before checking emails.
- Use a different bathroom at work.

See! It's simple to change your routine. However, I'm willing to bet this insignificant change feels strange.

If you stop after one day, your brain will take you right back to your old ways, even if the new routine makes sense! So you'll need to keep this change experiment going for a few days to fully appreciate how willing your brain is to accept it, but I think you get the gist. Plainly stated, we're not only habitual creatures but also highly adaptable ones.

Daily Result and Reflections: You did it! That good old report card is filling up! Go give yourself another check!

Self-Reflection: To change a habit, you must take hold of the reins and steer your brain in a new direction. With repetition, that new habit will take hold and feel like a perfect fit. However, change is initially uncomfortable.

For Karen, it took one week to start feeling the difference, but the discomfort was worthwhile. After 17 days without refined sugar, she noticed less inflammation, felt lighter, had more energy, and lost 10 pounds.

Discomfort accompanies change, even when the change improves your life. What did you change today? Record it in the space provided and describe how it felt.

_____

_____

_____

_____

_____

_____

"To change a habit, you must take hold of the reins and steer your brain in a new direction."

DAY 9

DON'T BEAT YOURSELF UP

Daily Focus: What has your body done for you today? A lot! Today, you set your focus on appreciating all of the amazing things your body is willing to do for you.

Daily Motivation: *Your Body Is a Well-Oiled Machine* I remember my first car. It was a sporty, little, light blue Toyota Celica. I took such good care of that car. I washed it a couple times a week, protected it from nicks, shined the wheels, and checked the oil. I loved that car and thought it was an engineering marvel. In reality, it was a 15-year-old rust bucket that had been in a major accident and leaked when it rained. I loved it not because of how it looked but because of what it did for me. It gave me freedom and took me places. In return, I gave it oil, fuel, and love.

Many people have fond memories of their first car and the feeling of pride that came with ownership. I wonder if most of us think about our bodies with such pride.

Without question, your body is an engineering marvel. When you keep it clean, protect it from nicks, and properly feed it, it gives you freedom and takes you places. But for one reason or another, it's common to dwell on the negative aspects of your body. Our criticisms are endless: The thighs are too fat, the midsection is flabby, some areas droop and others have bags, the legs are too short, the torso is too long, the ears are too big, and the eyes are too small.

You can't improve yourself if you don't believe what you have is worth improving. If you look in a mirror and only see faults, how does that impact how you care for your body? If you peer at your reflection and wish you could trade it in for a newer model, how does that influence your self-care efforts? If you hold on to a negative self-image, you'll be less inclined to maintain a healthy lifestyle and more inclined to do what's convenient and easy, going through life with a "who cares" attitude.

You might be thinking the opposite is true, worrying that by accepting your body as it is, you'll lose your desire to change. On the contrary, it will provide you with a new, stronger sense of self-worth, enhancing your drive to be your best.

John O'Leary's life offers a great example. In his book *On Fire: The 7 Choices to Ignite a Radically Inspired Life*, John shares how at the age of nine, he was burned on 100% of his body. As a curious boy, he wanted to see what would happen if he poured gasoline on a burning piece of cardboard. The blast that resulted was so powerful that it lifted him off his feet and slammed him against the garage wall. His parents were told his chance of survival was less than 1%. But after five months, dozens of surgeries, and the amputation of his fingers, John was wheeled out of the hospital. Despite the challenges, he not only survived, but he also thrived.

Fast-forward a couple decades. With visible scars and noticeably deformed hands, John became a hospital chaplain, helping families facing tragedy. He started rehabbing houses, turning his experience into a successful real estate development business, and today he's a highly sought-after inspirational speaker. He shares his life with his loving wife and their four children.

What if John had hidden from the world because of his deformities? What if he dwelled on the negative aspects of his body or waited until his scars were less visible to move on with his life?

Today, I'd like you to shift your focus away from perceived flaws to what your body does for you. You'll discover you don't have many friends as loyal as your body. Think about it. You've abused your body. We've all done it in one way or another—from feeding it processed food to not exercising it to subjecting it to high levels of stress. Sometimes, this abuse has gone on for decades, but your body is still willing to breathe for you 14 times a minute and pump blood throughout your body 100,000 times per day.

Your body is worth its weight in gold! Cherish it by treating it to a sugar-free day. Feed it nutritious whole foods so it can sustain a high energy level. Take it for regular walks and avoid damaging its interior with critical and self-defeating thoughts.

Daily Action: Appreciating Your Body

For today's action step, you'll soak in a little self-appreciation by listing five things you appreciate about your body. You don't need to choose things you like about your appearance, although those are fine to include. But also find things you like about how your body works and what it does for you. I want you to make your list specific to you, but to get you warmed up, here are a few examples:

- I'm so thankful I'm disease free.
- It's pretty cool having two working legs to get me around.
- I like my eyes.
- I'm so glad my feet are pain free.
- I appreciate that my body is strong enough to walk a mile.

Now it's your turn. List five things you appreciate about your body or yourself.

1. _____

2. _____

3. _____

4. _____

5. _____

If you find yourself becoming doubtful, negative, or cynical about your list, stop yourself. You can't prevent thoughts from entering your mind, but you can cut them short before they change how you feel about yourself.

Daily Result and Reflections: You did it! Go get that check on your "I Did It!" report card!

Self-Reflection: Think back through your day and jot down a few ways your body supported you. Did it keep breathing and pumping blood? Did it digest your food, carry you up a flight of stairs, let you see and hear what was going on around you? That's a pretty good friend, isn't it?

_____

_____

_____

_____

_____

_____

DAY 10

TAKE THE PATH LESS TRAVELED-YOUR OWN!

Daily Focus: It's easy to follow the crowd. But where is the crowd leading you? Today, you recommit to taking another step on your straight and narrow path to exceptional health.

Daily Motivation: *Following the Crowd* Do you ever feel as if the pursuit of health is nothing more than an adult version of follow the leader? Yesterday's fitness crazes were Zumba and Pilates. If you couldn't merengue yourself into shape or list the six essential Pilates principles, you felt like an outsider. Today, yoga and jujitsu are more likely to make you one of the cool kids.

Throughout a lifetime, we're exposed to many trends and fads, and most of us have followed the crowd a time or two. Unfortunately, following the crowd has its disadvantages.

When researchers looked at obesity trends, their findings suggested that obesity might be "socially contagious." They found that a person's risk of obesity went up by 57% if a friend became obese, 40% if a sibling did, and 37% if a spouse did.

Your commitment to completing *Zero Sugar / One Month* shows that you're willing to follow your own path and run your own race. You've chosen commitment over convenience and you'll reap the rewards. But I won't lie: The next few days will require your attention. With today being Day 10, you've officially entered the middle portion of your goal—*cue the yawn.*

Goals are journeys with exciting starts, exhilarating finishes, and mundane, just-get-through-it middles. The onset of a goal brings with it feelings of excitement and motivation. Those positive feelings are because of a rush of hormones, specifically dopamine and serotonin, that produces a feel-good sensation throughout your body. In other words, starting a goal feels great and you bask in a "*Let's do this*" motivating mindset for the first week or so. Unfortunately, this hormone high doesn't last. When it decreases, so does your motivation.

That motivation dip doesn't mean something has gone wrong with your plan. It's simply the way your physiology works. However, if you aren't aware of this phenomenon, you can give up on your goal or jump ship looking for the next plan because starting anew gives you a fresh hit of the feel-good hormones.

Those who study the goal achievement process identify predictable patterns in motivation and demotivation along the path to success. In other words, it is normal to think "*I've got this!*" on Monday and "*I'm frustrated*" on Thursday. The beauty is that doing the right thing for your body, even when you feel unmotivated, allows your brain to change and establish new patterns. With time, your new behaviors become self-sustaining, bringing your goal within reach. The thing to remember is it's normal to experience uncomfortable feelings when working toward a goal. Your job is to stay in the game.

Pat followed her own path to better health and reaped the rewards, losing a total of 54 pounds over the course of a year. While she sporadically practiced intermittent fasting, she credits the majority of her weight loss to getting serious about giving up sugar.

She never thought she could truly give up sugar and not be miserable, but today, it doesn't bother her one bit to sit next to someone eating one of her former favorite sweets. And the best part of her new lifestyle is no pain! She was nearly to the point of walking away from photographing weddings because by the end of an eight-hour wedding day, her joint and muscle pain was awful.

For Pat, mindset has been the key to staying on course. Instead of feeling sorry for herself that she "can't" have sugar, she's so thankful she now has the knowledge that's changing her health and giving her new life. At 52 years old, she runs literal circles around her 35-year-old former self.

Through *Zero Sugar / One Month*, you've already completed actions and used tools that are helping you stay in the game with less conscious thought. You've cleaned up your environment to keep tempting treats out of sight. You're using Stoppers to avoid unnecessary snacks and desserts, and you're eating whole food that stabilizes your blood sugar, preventing blood sugar crashes that drive cravings and fatigue.

Yes, you've entered the mundane middle period of your no-sugar month. But if you dig deep and stick to your commitment, I promise you that any struggle you face today will be long forgotten once you reach that glorious Day 30. I encourage you to stay the course and see your goal through. Aren't you curious about what will happen at the end of the 30 days? Close your eyes, picture that moment, and feel the joy build inside you as you realize you kept your commitment, faced the challenge head-on, and didn't back down!

Daily Action: Track Your Progress

Today, you'll retake the self-assessment to note your progress. Use the blank assessment sheets provided on pages 81 and 82 and then compare your answers to those you recorded on Day 0 (pg. 31).

Daily Result and Reflections: You did it! Another sugar-free day is in the bag! Flip back to page 13, fill in the Day 10 box on your report card, and give yourself a well-deserved pat on the back.

Self-Reflection: There's a reason you chose this sugar-free goal—a very important one. Recall that reason and record it below. Were you feeling depressed about your weight? Were you facing diabetes? Were you tired of always being tired? There was a strong desire to begin this journey. You don't want to trade your progress for a few brief moments of gratification, and you don't want to quit before the magic happens!

_____

_____

_____

_____

_____

_____

DAY 10 SELF-ASSESSMENT

Body Stats

Below, you'll find room to record your current body measurements. If you don't have access to all the measurements, simply record what you can.

Current Weight _____

Body Fat % _____

BMI _____

Fasting Blood Sugar _____

Measurements

Measure against bare skin. Use a flexible tape measure or a string you can later hold up to a ruler to determine your measurements.

Chest (measure around the fullest area) _____

Waist (measure one inch (2.5cm) above your belly button) _____

Hips (measure around the fullest area with your heels together) _____

Right Arm (measure around the fullest area above the elbow) _____

Right Thigh (measure around the fullest area) _____

Photos

Take selfies or ask a friend for help. Strike the same poses as you did on Day 0 (such as a full-body picture from the front, back, and side as well as a close-up of your face). For easy comparison, wear the same clothing for each photo session and stand in front of the same solid background.

Progress Chart

After filling in the Progress Chart below, compare your answers to those you gave on Day 0 (pg. 31).

NON-SCALE ASSESSMENT	TRUE	MOSTLY TRUE	(UNSURE) NEUTRAL	MOSTLY UNTRUE	NOT TRUE
My pants fit loose.					
My rings fit loose.					
My sleep is restful.					
My ability to focus is strong.					
My energy level is high.					
My sugar cravings are low.					
My joints are pain-free.					
My ability to cope with stress is high.					
My outlook is positive.					
My nose is rarely stuffy.					
I do not snore at night.					
My skin is clear of blemishes.					
There is no swelling in my legs.					
My sense of accomplishment is high.					

"Doing the right thing for your body, even when you feel unmotivated, allows your brain to change and establish new patterns."

DAYS 11-20

A Sneak Peek at the Key Points Ahead

Day 11: Making a choice feels uncomfortable but opens the door to opportunity.

Day 12: We all hear ANTs (automatic negative thoughts). Acknowledge them and let them go.

Day 13: If you look, there's always something that went well.

Day 14: There are two types of hunger: true hunger and false hunger. True hunger requires food, whereas false hunger requires understanding.

Day 15 Don't stop before the magic happens!

Day 16: Up your game by avoiding the "elimination trifecta": sugar, flour, and seed oils.

Day 17: Drop the self-judgment and get curious.

Day 18: Fear and panic are false motivators. It's your hard work and commitment that have made the difference.

Day 19: Goals are reached one day at a time.

Day 20: There's still work to be done, but for today, you're okay.

DAY 11

MAKE THE CHOICE

Daily Focus: Avoiding sugar is a choice. Making that choice feels uncomfortable, but it unlocks a world of opportunities.

Daily Motivation: *Opportunity Cost* When I was 12 years old, I decided to become an Olympic gold medal gymnast because I had watched the Olympics, and I saw those girls and thought, "*Gee, that must be so cool to be like them.*" But then I realized those athletes had to eat special diets, live apart from their families, and spend hours in the gym every day. I didn't want to do those things, but I sure did want that medal!

Not surprisingly, I never made it to the Olympics. It wasn't because I lacked athletic ability. It was because I made a mistake in my thinking. I thought that because I'd decided that being an Olympian was a *cool idea*, I'd also made the *choice* to do so. These are two entirely different things. There's one very important factor that separates a good idea from a choice: opportunity cost.

You see, when I was 12, I wanted the opportunity to be an Olympic athlete, but I wasn't willing to pay the cost. Opportunity cost is based on the realization that we have countless opportunities in life—so many that we can't possibly pursue them all. Therefore, for every new opportunity that we accept, such as maintaining a healthy weight, there's another opportunity we must let go of, such as eating refined foods.

This is where most of us go wrong. We don't want to make a choice. We want to keep eating unhealthy foods *and* live a healthy, vibrant life at our ideal weight. In fact, we're willing to spend years pursuing this elusive, magical solution. I can attest to this personally.

One of my earliest memories is of riding home on the school bus and day-dreaming about the sugary treats waiting for me when I walked through the door. I'd also hope no one would be in the kitchen so I could grab and dash with my candy bar and cookies, devouring them in peace—just me and my sugar.

My obsession with eating sugar wasn't only an internal struggle—it also showed on the outside. In high school, I started gaining weight, which led to a summer of eating lettuce and nothing but lettuce. That crash diet in my teens caused me to lose weight, but because I'd taken the weight off in a way that couldn't be sustained, it came back on as soon as I returned to my old eating pattern.

I began yo-yo dieting and my weight roller-coastered up and down with each attempt. I stayed in that cycle because I never made a full and clear choice to stop eating sugar. In fact, I approached it from the opposite end of the spectrum.

Every time I started another sugarless period, I looked at it as a temporary punishment. It was something I had to do so I could get my weight down and get back to my fun foods. The thought of actually living sugar-free never even entered my mind. I couldn't imagine a life without my junk food, which by that point felt more like a comforting friend than food.

Over the next couple decades, I wrestled with myself, yo-yoing back and forth between sugar and dieting. Nothing changed until I *chose* to let go of the thing that was preventing permanent weight control.

When I stopped looking at giving up sugar as an annoying temporary fix and instead made a choice to cut the sugar, I was given the opportunity to live in a healthy body. And something unbelievable happened: I began to enjoy food even more! No longer were my taste buds dulled by the intense sweetness of sugar. This allowed me to thoroughly enjoy the subtle sweetness of berries, nuts, and other natural foods.

Making a choice is scary because it leads you into an uncertain future. However, I assure you that life is so much better on the other side of sugar. There's less bloating, less time spent in the bathroom, less unavoidable napping, and less craziness.

Daily Action: Choosing Sugar-Free

Take a moment to read through the comments below. Notice the benefits that came into these individuals' lives once they made the choice to stop eating sugar.

Catt discovered that the less sugar she ate, the less she wanted sugary foods.

Helen experienced renewed energy when she eliminated all sweet and processed foods. She now enjoys shopping for healthy foods as well as planning and preparing meals.

Isaac was thrilled to discover that the fatigue he used to experience was gone two months after going sugar-free. He found that his mood stabilized and his body felt more at peace.

Ivana lost 15 pounds (7 kilograms) in three months by following a low-carb, low-sugar diet and practicing intermittent fasting. She's now more mindful of what she eats and is benefitting from a calmer stomach, more flexibility, and clearer skin.

Keith described the feeling of no longer needing to devour sweets without a thought as freeing.

You can see from these experiences that many opportunities open up when you move away from sugar (such as fewer cravings, more energy, enjoyable shopping and food prep, less fatigue, stable moods, weight loss, less stomach discomfort, more flexibility, clearer skin, and freedom). Jot down a few things that jumped out at you and made you say "Yes, that's something I want!"

_____

_____

_____

_____

_____

_____

Daily Result and Reflections: You did it! Go to page 13 and record another day in the books!

Self-Reflection: Making a choice to give up sugar can feel like losing a friend, bringing up negative emotions like sadness, fear, and mournfulness. However, sugar is a toxic friend leading you down the wrong path. It's time to formally break up with sugar. Use the space below to write down a few words you'd like to say to sugar or to write out a full breakup letter telling sugar how it deceives you, zaps your energy, and muddles your thinking.

_____

_____

_____

_____

_____

_____

_____

_____

_____

_____

_____

_____

_____

_____

_____

_____

_____

_____

_____

_____

_____

_____

_____

DAY 12

EXTERMINATING ANTS

Daily Focus: One thing can always be said about sugar: You never wake up wishing you'd eaten more of it the night before. Today, you are making the conscious decision to stop overthinking and just do it!

Daily Motivation: *Just Do It! vs. Just Get It Over With!* One of Nike's most famous advertising slogans is "Just Do It!" It seems the whole world has grabbed hold of this pithy little phrase. The appeal is its simplicity—three short words that pack a powerful call to action. Stop thinking, planning, and contemplating—and just do it!

Hump day (Day 15) is just three days away. Seeing that halfway point in your grasp is lifting your spirits and you're seeing glimpses of the awesomeness of getting sugar out of your diet. But you're also experiencing the *"Are we there yet?"* blues that come with the middle of any goal. You're probably not jumping out of bed with the phrase *"Just do it"* resounding in your head. In fact, you might be dragging yourself out of bed, grabbing a cup of coffee, and proclaiming *"Just get it over with."* Admittedly, that saying doesn't pack the power the Nike message does.

It's a common misconception that people who regularly eat a healthy diet love every moment of it. This isn't true. Some days, it's more of a chore than a delight. However, one thing can always be said about sugar: You never wake up the next morning thinking, *"I'm so glad I ate sugar last night."* The trick is getting to the next morning without giving in to temptation. To do that, you must be able to recognize and exterminate ANTs.

Dr. Daniel Amen, psychiatrist and author of *Change Your Brain, Change Your Life*, coined the term ANTs in the early 1990s. It's an acronym that stands for Automatic Negative Thoughts. ANTs are extremely common, crawling through the head of anyone who sets a goal to change.

Many people find it easy to declare a goal but fall short of reaching it because of fears and doubts. Maybe you've experienced this in the past. You write down or even just think about a goal, and suddenly, you feel a wave of discomfort wash over you. This can happen even if you have a strong desire to make a positive change in your life. What happened was your brain got invaded by ANTs. These pesky little thoughts show up because part of you feels uncomfortable about change, taking action, or the goal itself.

Do any of these thoughts sound familiar?

- Living without sugar will be a lot of work and too stressful.
- Even if I succeed, my friends will keep eating sugar. I'm going to miss out on the fun.
- I've never been able to do this in the past. What makes me think I can do it now?
- It's not fair I have this problem!

ANTs can be bold (*"I don't think I can do it."*) or sneaky and conniving (*"I'm too tired to worry about sugar today. Shouldn't I allow myself a little happiness?"*).

Regardless of how they show up, you can be sure that when you start to hear them running around inside your head, you're somehow associating the process of reaching your goal (or the outcome of that goal) with discomfort, displeasure, or pain.

Tip Jar

It's good to note that ANTs don't show up to make your life miserable. They pop up to protect you from the uncertainty that comes with change. So there's no reason to get upset with them. Just know they're an expected pest everyone deals with. This acknowledgment is often enough to quiet them.

Daily Action: Exterminating ANTs

Here's a three-step process to exterminate ANTs.

1. Hear the ANT.
2. Acknowledge that ANTs are expected pests that everyone deals with.
3. Let go of the ANT by shifting your focus.

Giving automatic negative thoughts your focus does you no good. If you think about the ANTs crawling around in your head, you'll notice they're often attempting to predict the future. But no one can predict the future. It must be experienced.

When you hear an ANT, acknowledge that it's a normal and expected pest. This simple acknowledgment robs it of its power. You can then let go of the negative thought because that's all it is—a thought. It's not a physical part of you, so it's not attached to you in any way. Therefore, whenever you feel ready, shift your focus to something else. When you do, you'll feel freer, lighter, and more capable.

There are countless ways to quickly shift your focus. Here are just a few:

- Look around you and consciously notice something. "*Those flowers are beautiful!*"
- Recall your "Big Why." "*I love being able to fit comfortably in my clothes.*"
- Turn on some favorite music or listen to a podcast or audiobook.
- Remind yourself that today is the only day that needs your attention. ANTs are nothing more than a poor attempt at predicting the future.
- Plaster a smile on your face. This fake-it-until-you-make-it method of shifting your focus works! Give it a try!

Daily Result and Reflections: You did it! Wahoo! Flip back to page 13 and fill in the Day 12 box on your "I Did It!" report card.

Self-Reflection: If you dwell on an ANT, it will grow in strength, threatening to derail your goal. The trick is to shift your focus away from it.

Write down an ANT you heard today.

_____

_____

_____

_____

How did you (or could you) shift your focus to squash the little pest?

_____

_____

_____

_____

THAT WENT WELL

Daily Focus: There is more than one way to look at any situation, and you get to choose your focus. Today, you are directing your focus toward the good of life by acknowledging what went well.

Daily Motivation: *Have a "That Went Well" Day* "According to the weight chart, I should be a little bit taller." I first heard this tongue-in-cheek saying years ago. While it's a facetious statement, it points out that there's more than one way to look at a situation: You're not overweight—you're undertall.

Yesterday, you learned that ANTs (automatic negative thoughts) are goal disruptors that pop into your head. When you focus on them, they cloud your judgment and erode your determination to change. Fortunately, ANTs can be exterminated by replacing them with helpful thoughts that allow you to see any situation more accurately and positively.

Remember that just having a gloomy thought isn't detrimental. It's only when that thought is allowed to linger that it gains strength and grows. To get rid of an ANT before it does damage, hear it, acknowledge it, and let go of it by directing your focus toward a positive thought. The neat thing is that even the slightest shift can turn your attitude around, allowing you to feel better quickly.

For example, it's easy to get upset about little things in life. The coffee pot is empty; the dog won't stop barking; your computer updates are taking too long. If you focus on these things, you get irritated and might get tempted to take the edge off with a little something sweet. We're all guilty of this. However, what we fail to see is that in those same moments, there are good things happening. Today, you'll put another tool in your ANT extermination toolbox by giving yourself a "That went well" day.

This focal shift is not pie-in-the-sky positive thinking or even being grateful for the blessing in your life. It requires you to acknowledge the little things that are good but often overlooked. For example, when you get a pull-through parking space in a crowded parking lot, say "That went well." When your dog goes outside and doesn't get her leash wrapped around the patio chair like she usually would, say "That went well." When the mailman brings you a check instead of a bill, say "That went well."

Tip Jar

Take your "that went well" acknowledgment to the next level by doing it as a preemptive exercise. When you feel like complaining, ask yourself: "What is going well?" You'll always be able to come up with something that puts a positive spin on the situation.

Daily Action: Acknowledging What Went Well

Today, I encourage you to give yourself a "That went well" day, putting emphasis on what's going well with your health and eating.

> When the salad you reluctantly order at the restaurant turns out to be delicious, say: *"That went well!"*

> When you cut open an avocado and it is the perfect ripeness, say: *"That went well."*

> When you realize no one even blinked an eye when you passed on the cupcakes, say: *"That went well."*

> When your Stopper allows you to comfortably avoid dessert, say: *"That went well."*

> When a friend says you're looking good, reply with a verbal thank you and a silent *"That went well."*

Mental exercises like this take conscious effort, but when you do them, you wipe out the subtle emotional eating triggers that cause you to act in ways that don't support your goal.

Daily Result and Reflections: You did it! That went well! Now go get that check mark!

Self-Reflection: When it comes to eating, no one's perfect. If you focus on imperfections, you'll quickly get discouraged. However, if you do the opposite and focus on what you did right, your confidence will build, helping you move toward a happy, healthy, sugar-free life. Think back through your day and record what went well.

_____

_____

_____

_____

_____

_____

"Knowing the difference between true and false hunger allows you to make better eating decisions and achieve long-term health and weight control."

FEED TRUE HUNGER, IGNORE FALSE HUNGER

Daily Focus: True hunger is driven by your body's physiological need for fuel, whereas false hunger is driven by other factors, such as habits, routines, whims, and scarcity. Today's hunger scale exercise gives you the tool to tell the difference.

Daily Motivation: *Is That True or False Hunger?* Today marks two weeks without sugar and your dedication has paid off. Even if you've had a slip or two along the way, by this point, your physiology has changed from relying mainly on sugar and carbs for energy to relying more on fat. Burning fat is like burning logs on a fire. It takes a while to get them lit, but once they're burning, they supply a steady stream of energy and hunger control. However, that doesn't mean you won't *feel* hungry.

You see, there are two types of hunger we must deal with: true hunger and false hunger. True hunger is driven by your body's physiological need for fuel. But even when true hunger is satisfied, false hunger can remain. That's because false hunger is driven by extraneous factors, such as habits, routines, whims, and scarcity.

Knowing the difference between true and false hunger allows you to make better eating decisions and achieve long-term health and weight control. However, if you're like many people, you've lost your ability to distinguish one from the other.

We often decide to eat based on external cues, such as an enticing TV commercial, the smell of a favorite food, or the time of day (*"It is noon. I should eat lunch."*). When you base your decision to eat on these factors, you pay little attention to how much your body wants or needs the food. In other words, external cues make you feel like eating even if you're not truly hungry.

Fortunately, there's a simple exercise that will restore your ability to tell the difference between true and false.

Daily Action: Rate Your Hunger

Today, you'll learn how to rate your hunger using a hunger scale.

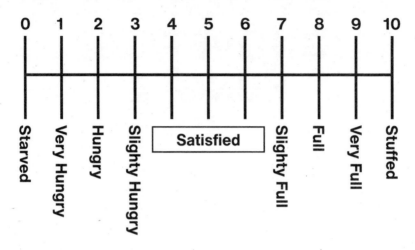

Note that the Hunger Scale runs from 0 to 10, with "0" meaning you're starving and "10" meaning you're stuffed. Think of your hunger level as you would the gas tank of your car. When your tank is nearing empty, you need to refuel. When it's full, you don't.

The scale itself is simple. But you might find it surprisingly hard to pinpoint where you land on the scale at any given moment. It's a skill many of us have lost.

To bridge that learning gap for you, let me give you some prompts:

- You're at 10 if you're uncomfortably full or need to unbutton your pants.
- You're at 9 if you forced yourself to eat everything on your plate despite knowing it would push you over the edge.
- You're at 8 if you just ate a big meal but feel comfortable.
- You're at 7 if a couple hours have passed since your big meal or you just had a lighter meal.
- You're at 4, 5, or 6 if your body feels comfortable, your energy is good, and eating doesn't feel like a pressing matter. This is the satisfied range and where you'll feel the most comfortable.

- You're at 3 if hunger just popped into your head but you don't feel an immediate need to eat.

- You're at 2 if hunger is annoying but manageable. This is a common level to be at a half hour before lunch or dinner. You know you can wait, but you're happy mealtime is around the corner.

- You're at 1 if hunger is distracting you or you're feeling low on energy, lightheaded, *hangry*, or having trouble concentrating on your work.

- You're at 0 if hunger has completely hijacked your brain. You can't focus on anything other than food.

You don't have to wait until you are at 0 to eat. For example, if you're at 3 and you're meeting someone for lunch. You can certainly eat, but knowing you're a 3 will help you make better food choices or help you feel confident you can eat a lighter meal and walk away feeling comfortable. If you're at 1 or 2 and it's a couple hours before mealtime, consider having a snack or something to drink. (Thirst can mimic hunger.)

If you find you have the desire to eat, but when you rate your hunger, you fall at 7 or above, your body doesn't need food. This is false hunger and it's likely being driven by an external cue, habit, or even scarcity, such as thinking "*It's the last serving on the tray. If I don't eat it now, I'll miss out.*"

Throughout the day, take time to rate your hunger. I encourage you to check your hunger level every two hours or at least immediately before each meal.

Use the chart below to record your hunger readings. You'll notice a space for adding notes. Use that space to record anything you feel might have influenced your hunger level. For example:

- I'm feeling stressed, happy, busy, etc.
- I've been fasting for 14 hours.
- I'm at work, a restaurant, the grocery store, etc.

My Hunger Record

TIME	HUNGER #	NOTES

Tip Jar

Record your hunger numbers for the next five days and you'll see patterns emerge. For example, you might notice regular times during the day when you're tempted to eat but not physically hungry. This newfound knowledge will help you make better eating decisions effortlessly.

Daily Result and Reflections: You did it! Your report card is filling up!

Self-Reflection: Stress, anxiety, busyness, uncertainty, and loneliness are just some of the factors that cause us to feel like eating when we're not truly hungry. Review the notes you added to the chart above or reflect on your day. Was there a time you thought your hunger number would be higher or lower than it was? What was going on that might have been driving false hunger?

_____

_____

_____

_____

HUNGER-SATISFYING SALAD

A daily salad is a great strategy for healthy living. The non-starchy vegetables fill your stomach and the addition of hunger-satisfying fats and protein keeps hunger away for hours. Here's my favorite daily salad.

SERVES: 1

2–4 cups (about 128g) mixed salad greens

2 tbsp feta cheese crumbles

½ avocado, chopped

½ small (50g) apple, chopped

1 tbsp raw sunflower seeds

1 tbsp chopped walnuts

1 tbsp raw pumpkin seeds

2 tbsp full-fat salad dressing

Place the salad greens in a serving bowl. Add the remaining ingredients and enjoy!

Notes:

For an even heartier salad, add additional fat/protein choices, such as salmon, chicken, steak, or hard-boiled eggs. Vegetarian additions include lentils, beans, and additional nuts and seeds.

Many low-fat salad dressings contain sugar or high-fructose corn syrup. Look for a full-fat dressing made with avocado or olive oil or make your own at home by blending olive oil and balsamic vinegar. Use 3 tablespoons of oil for each tablespoon of vinegar and give your homemade dressing a kick by adding Dijon mustard, salt, pepper, or chopped herbs, such as basil, parsley, or thyme.

NUTRITION PER SERVING

| Calories 494 | Carbohydrates 23.8g | Sugars 8.2g |
| Fat 42.1g | Fiber 9g | Protein 12.1g |

"Keep your commitment to avoiding sugar high on your priority list— and don't stop before the magic happens!"

DON'T STOP BEFORE THE MAGIC HAPPENS!

Daily Focus: You are halfway there! Hooray! Don't stop before the magic happens!

Daily Motivation: *Priorities* Years ago, I was the hapless recipient of a rock hitting my windshield. That rock left a small but inconveniently placed crack in the glass. Being a college student at the time—and finances were tight, to say the least—I never bothered to get the crack fixed. It was simply never a priority. But the crack bothered me. It was at such a place that you couldn't drive the car without having to look through it. It frustrated me every time I got behind the steering wheel. It embarrassed me every time I'd take a passenger for a ride. I kept thinking that one of these days, I'd do something about that crack, but weeks became months, months turned into years, and the crack remained.

Lifestyle diseases are conditions that can potentially be prevented or reversed through diet and lifestyle changes. They include diabetes, cardiovascular disease, and obesity. These disorders are like cracks in your windshield. It's frustrating to think our habits are contributing to health problems. However, because of the pressures of work, family, activities, and countless other life events, fixing them never seems to move up on the priority list.

When you started your *Zero Sugar* month, I bet the timing wasn't ideal. But you did start, and today, you find yourself at the halfway point! But even though you're cresting hump day, your mind might still be working overtime, trying to convince you to come to your senses and unwind with some ice cream already!

You can't wait for temptations to go away. The irony is that the only thing that will lessen the temptation to eat sugar is not giving in to it. And the longer you go without sugar, the more your taste buds and brain chemistry reset, loosening sugar's grip on your life. In other words, make this moment the time you fix the crack! Keep your commitment to avoiding sugar high on your priority list—and don't stop before the magic happens!

For Maryellen, that magic happened and had staying power. A self-declared sugar addict, she decided to give up sugar and all sweeteners for a month. She started on a Friday and that first weekend was rough. However, the ill feeling lifted and she stuck with her sugar-free commitment for 30 days. Soon after, she had one treat at a family get-together and felt so poorly afterward that she decided to return to her no-sweets diet. That was almost eight years ago. She has no regrets about getting off the sugar roller coaster, and today, it doesn't bother her at all to skip the cakes and cookies because she knows now what they were doing to her.

Daily Action: Recharge Your Commitment

For today's action step, you'll soak in the good feeling of accomplishment. Sit in a comfortable chair and look ahead two weeks from today. See yourself crossing that *Zero Sugar* finish line. Doesn't it feel good? Really put yourself there, allowing the joyful sensation to fill your chest and spread through your body. What are you seeing?

Are you celebrating the number on the scale?

Are you beaming as you look in the mirror with the confidence of knowing "*you did it!*"?

Are you in awe of what you can do when you put your mind to it?

As you learned on Day 6, true motivation comes from within and it's your emotions that pull that motivation to the surface. This exercise only takes 1 minute to complete, so do it a few times throughout the day to resurface your motivation.

Daily Result and Reflections: You did it! Halfway is in the bag. That deserves a big, beautiful mark on your "I Did It!" report card.

Self-Reflection: That crack in my car windshield was annoying, but at the time, I was willing to give up a clear view to focus on school. Health is a different issue. Poor diet and lifestyle choices adversely affect your energy level, mood, and disease risk. In this hectic world, it's easy to push health down on the priority list. But you can't outrun the consequences of a poor diet. Isn't it nice to know that for today, you still have a choice? Use the space below to record your thoughts at this halfway point. Regular journaling reinforces your new, healthy lifestyle and reminds you about how far you've come.

_____

_____

_____

_____

_____

_____

"The safest way to avoid harmful ingredients is to cook at home and avoid fast-food and prepackaged meals."

DAY 16

THE ELIMINATION TRIFECTA

Daily Focus: Today, you are taking the opportunity to up your game by avoiding the Elimination Trifecta—sugar, flour, and seed oils.

Daily Motivation: *Opt for Optimum Health* Do you want to hit your new healthy lifestyle out of the park? There are three foods to avoid, which I call the "elimination trifecta." You already know the negative health consequences of eating sugar. What might not be on your radar are flour and seed oils.

Flour is made by grinding down different plants. The white flour we're most familiar with is made by grinding grains. But flour can also be made from other plant foods, such as almonds and coconut, giving us almond flour and coconut flour. These more natural flour varieties have a nutritional edge over white flour and don't produce the same dramatic spikes in blood sugar and insulin. However, swapping them for white flour so you can keep baked snacks and desserts in your diet will make it very hard to control hunger and cravings.

Seed oils (aka vegetable oils) are problematic in many ways. Most of these refined oils are high in inflammatory omega-6 fatty acids and can be manipulated to give us trans fats. Also, the oil is hard to extract from the plant and must be pulled out using harmful chemicals or heat that causes the oil to degrade.

Unfortunately, seed oils are cheap, so they're the oils restaurants and packaged food companies typically use and the least expensive option at the grocery store. Soybean oil is the most commonly used seed oil, but there are many others, as you'll see listed in the chart below.

Daily Action: Become a Food Detective

I invite you to become a food detective, looking out for the elimination trifecta. This job isn't simple because there are so many different types of sugars, flours, and seed oils. The chart below provides a list of alternate names.

To complete today's action step, avoid any packaged food with a type of sugar, flour, or seed oil listed in the first three ingredients.

─────────────── **SUGAR** ───────────────

- Agave
- Corn syrup
- Dextrose
- Fructose

- Fruit juice concentrate
- Glucose
- Honey
- Lactose

- Maltodextrin
- Maltose
- Molasses
- Sucrose
- Syrup

Note: At this point, noncaloric sugar substitutes are allowed. However, you'll be asked to remove them from your diet for the final week. For a full list of added sugars and sweeteners, see the FAQ (pg. 18).

─────────────── **FLOUR** ───────────────

- All-purpose (white) flour
- Almond flour
- Buckwheat flour
- Chickpea flour
- Coconut flour

- Corn flour
- Gluten-free flour
- Oat flour
- Rye flour
- Semolina flour

- Spelt flour
- Tapioca flour (starch)
- Wheat flour
- Whole wheat flour

Note: If a food has flour listed as one of the first three ingredients, don't eat it, even if it's almond or coconut flour. A small amount is okay, but the food is too refined when flour is a primary ingredient.

SEED OILS

- Canola oil
- Corn oil
- Cottonseed oil
- Grapeseed oil

- Hydrogenated oil
- Peanut oil
- Rice bran oil
- Safflower oil

- Soybean oil
- Sunflower oil
- Vegetable oil

Note: You'll find acceptable oils and cooking fats on the food list (pg. 23).

No time to consult a list? I get it. Not everyone has time to become a food detective. You can accomplish today's action step without a list by cooking at home and sticking with whole foods.

Here's a sample menu:

Breakfast: Omelet (stuff with sauteed vegetables, meat, and/or cheese)

Lunch: Salad (top with chicken, salmon, or hard-boiled eggs) (vegetarian salad toppers: avocado, nuts, and seeds) (Try my Hunger-Satisfying Salad on page 101.)

Dinner: Meat, Fish, or Poultry (with a side of cooked, non-starchy vegetables) (Need quick recipes? Try my 30-Minute Dinner Plan on page 111.)

 Tip Jar

Vegetarian Dinner: Getting enough protein is a daily challenge for those who follow a plant-based diet. Vegetarian foods that contain protein include beans, lentils, nuts, quinoa, seeds, seitan, spirulina, tempeh, and tofu.

Tip Jar

When it comes to picking an oil to use in food prep, quality matters. Here are some terms to help you choose wisely.

Extra virgin means the oil is from the first extraction. This is beneficial because the first pressing contains more antioxidants and beneficial compounds than regular oil.

Cold-pressed or expeller-pressed describe ways oil is squeezed from a plant. The benefit of these two methods is they don't use nutrient-damaging heat or chemicals to extract the oil.

High oleic is a term associated with certain oils, including sunflower and safflower oil. Despite being seed oils, they contain a good amount of heart-healthy monounsaturated fat. While the overall health benefit of these oils is inconclusive, high oleic oils are better choices than other variations of the oils.

Daily Result and Reflections: You did it! Go get that check on your report card and give yourself an extra pat on the back if you eliminated the trifecta today!

Self-Reflection: The safest way to avoid harmful ingredients is to cook at home and avoid fast-food and prepackaged meals. Cooking is a valuable skill that saves money and improves your health. Reflect on home cooking for a moment. Is there anything that holds you back from doing it? What could you do to increase the number of meals you prepare at home?

_____

_____

_____

_____

_____

_____

30-Minute Dinner Plan

CHILI LIME CHICKEN TENDERS

Place the ingredients in a resealable plastic bag, shake them up, and put them on a baking sheet in the oven. In less than 30 minutes, you'll have this no-sugar, family-friendly entrée on the table!

SERVES: 4 · SERVING SIZE: 4 OUNCES (113g)

1 ½ tbsp avocado oil
1 ½ tbsp freshly squeezed
   lime juice
½ tbsp chili powder
½ tbsp smoked or regular paprika

½ tsp fine sea salt
¼ tsp ground
   black pepper
¼ tsp crushed red pepper
1 lb (454g) chicken tenderloins

1. Preheat the oven to 400°F (200°C). Line a rimmed baking sheet with aluminum foil or parchment paper and spray with nonstick cooking spray. Set aside.

2. Place the oil, lime juice, chili powder, paprika, salt, pepper, and crushed red pepper in a large resealable plastic bag. Smush the ingredients with your fingers to blend them.

3. Rinse the chicken tenderloins, pat dry with paper towels, and place them in the bag. Seal the bag and smush again to coat the chicken.

4. Arrange the tenders on the prepared sheet and bake for 15–17 minutes or until the chicken reaches an internal temperature of 165°F (74°C).

Note: You can boost the flavor by marinating the chicken tenderloins in the oil and spices overnight or for a few hours before cooking.

NUTRITION PER SERVING

Calories 249	Carbohydrates 1.6g	Sugars 0.3g
Fat 10.5g	Fiber 0.7g	Protein 35.4g

GARLIC MASHED CAULIFLOWER

This creamy and quick side dish is a flavorful low-starch substitution for mashed potatoes.

SERVES: 4 · **SERVING SIZE:** ¼ OF THE RECIPE

1lb (454g) fresh or frozen
cauliflower florets
⅓ cup (80g) full-fat mayonnaise
2 tbsp chicken broth
½ tsp freshly squeezed
lemon juice

½ tsp garlic powder
½ tsp fine sea salt
¼ tsp ground black pepper
2 tsp dried chives

1. In a large microwave-safe bowl, combine the cauliflower florets, mayonnaise, broth, lemon juice, garlic powder, salt, and pepper. Stir to lightly coat the florets.

2. Microwave on high for 12–13 minutes. You want the florets to be very tender and easily break apart with light pressure. Increase the cooking time by a couple minutes if you're using frozen cauliflower.

3. Place the cooked mixture in a food processor and blend until smooth.

4. Transfer the cauliflower mash to a serving bowl and fold in the chives before serving.

Note: The cauliflower can be cooked on the stove. Bring 1 cup of water to a boil in a medium-sized saucepan over high heat. Add the cauliflower florets and return to a boil. Stir, cover, and lower temperature to medium to simmer until the florets are tender. Place the cooked cauliflower and the remaining ingredients except the chives in the food processor. Blend until smooth and fold in the chives.

NUTRITION PER SERVING

Calories 165	Carbohydrates 6.4g	Sugars 2.3g
Fat 16.3g	Fiber 2.4g	Protein 2.5g

"Cooking is a valuable skill that saves money and improves your health."

SHIFT YOUR PERSPECTIVE

Daily Focus: Situations are not under your control, but how you view them is. Today, you turn any frown upside down by choosing curiosity over self-judgment.

Daily Motivation: *Enjoy the Journey* Hersheypark is nicknamed the Sweetest Place on Earth—not only because of its ties to the Hershey chocolate bar but also because it's a fun place to visit. Living a short drive from the park is, indeed, a treat, and when my daughter was little, we visited often, soaking in the pleasant atmosphere.

One particularly hot August day, I sat on a park bench to rest for a few moments while my daughter cooled off under the park's water sprinklers. As I glanced around at the crowd, I took notice of a young employee. The fact that he was part of the cleanup crew was obvious because he was dressed in an official park uniform and carried a small trash collector and broom. I was taken by the sullen expression on his face and the slowness of his actions as time after monotonous time, he'd spot a piece of trash and sweep it into the receptacle. I thought to myself: "I bet he doesn't think Hersheypark is the sweetest place on Earth."

Do you ever feel like you've been assigned to the cleanup crew? Do you know there's a wonderful, exciting world all around you, but you're so overwhelmed by the task set before you that you can't enjoy it?

Pursuing health might leave you feeling this way. You might think you're so out of shape, your eating habits are so poor, or you have so much weight to lose that happiness is a long way away. However, you don't have to be at your goal before you can enjoy life. The secret is in learning to enjoy the journey. How? By linking pleasure with things that would typically be associated with pain.

For example, let's consider our teenage employee. His unhappiness stemmed from the fact that he was linking his job to boredom. He could change that association by learning to link the cleanup crew to something important to himself as a young man. For example, he could view his job as one that can be performed at his own pace, giving him time to check out the teenage girls in the park. Adopting that new viewpoint could be enough to change his perspective from *"This job is so boring"* to *"This is a great job!"*

Now let's apply this to your pursuit of health. If you link the avoidance of sugar to pain and deprivation, shift your perspective. For example, you could focus on how eliminating sugar speeds weight loss and leads to pain-free joints. That's a nice payoff and all you have to do is avoid one ingredient, leaving many delicious foods still on the table.

Tip Jar

Try this perspective shift with any limiting belief you might be holding on to. With a willing spirit, you'll discover a whole new world around you. Let's try it with exercise. Do you link exercise to soreness and exhaustion? Why not link it to feeling alive? A daily workout can give you a sense of accomplishment. How would it feel to fully embrace life instead of letting it happen to you?

Daily Action: Get Curious

Become an observer of your life. One of the best ways to gain a new perspective on things is to step back from your situation and watch yourself as if you were watching someone else. Often, you're too close to the problem to see any possible solution. When you step back, you become a curious observer and find new ways of coping.

Curiosity is a true friend of anyone working toward a goal. It's simply learning how to ask yourself nonjudgmental questions so you can uncover the real reason for your actions.

To complete today's action step, actively swap criticism for curiosity. This requires you to pay attention to your internal dialogue. When it takes a negative turn, drop the self-judgment and get curious. For example, let's say you go overboard with a snack. Instead of beating yourself up, ask yourself why you felt a need to eat. This intentional curiosity allows your mind to stay open, keeps you calm, and prevents you from mindlessly repeating the behavior.

Example: You ate the home-baked treats in the breakroom.

> Why did you want to give in to the temptation? *"I felt like I was missing out by not eating the snack."*
>
> What was going on that made you question your no-sugar commitment? *"Everyone around me was grabbing the treats. It made me feel left out."*
>
> What could you do differently next time? *"I could store my favorite tea in the breakroom and busy myself with preparing and sipping it. This will allow me to socialize and stay true to my commitment."*

Daily Result and Reflections: You did it! Another sugar-free day is in the bag!

Self-Reflection: Before starting *Zero Sugar / One Month*, eating sugar was what you knew. It felt comfortable and you might have even attached advantages to it: It's fun. It gives you an energy boost. It makes you normal. However, continuing to defend sugar is like digging to get out of a hole. You convince yourself you're doing the right thing, but in reality, you're making matters worse. You can't change conditioned thinking if you're unaware it exists. Take a moment to consider how you view sugar. Are there ways you defend it or attach advantages to it? Simply writing them down shines a light on them, helping you leave them in the past.

_____

_____

_____

_____

_____

_____

"You don't have to be at your goal before you can enjoy life. The secret is in learning to enjoy the journey."

CONSISTENT EFFORT MATTERS

Daily Focus: You are still in the game, proving that you've got what it takes to see this challenge through. Today, you acknowledge the new, enjoyable healthy habits you've developed.

Daily Motivation: *What's Your Health Plan Built Out Of?* The three little pigs decided to get in shape.

The first little pig built his health plan out of panic. He realized he had only a few weeks to shape up before the swimming hole opened for the summer and he hadn't shed the extra pounds he'd put on over the winter. In a panic, he decided to go on a five-day fast.

The second little pig built his plan out of fear. His doctor told him his blood sugar was too high, and if he did not get it under control, he risked developing diabetes. He was afraid. He didn't want health problems and knew it was time for a complete lifestyle overhaul. He immediately changed his diet, gave up caffeine, and joined the local gym, committing to an hour of exercise each day.

The third little pig built his health plan out of desire. He acknowledged he needed to lose 10 pounds. He realized this was important to him because he wanted the energy and good feelings that come with following healthy habits. He sat down and devised a sensible plan that reduced his calorie intake by swapping sugary snacks for healthy options. He also started walking in the morning and stopped eating after dinner.

After two days without food, the first little pig was hungry and irritable. He decided fasting was a bad idea and quit.

By the end of the first week, the second little pig was depressed, tired, and overwhelmed by all the changes. He decided this was no way to go through life and let temptation win out. He quit before the second week began.

The third little pig revisited his goals each morning. He committed to following his plan for the day and not worrying about tomorrow. He had some hard times but stayed on course, knowing that consistent effort would pay off. He felt more in control with each passing day and celebrated as the scale showed a lower number each week.

Before long, the third pig had reached his goal and felt great! He was proud of his accomplishment and felt confident he could maintain his new healthy lifestyle. The other two pigs were preparing to start a new diet they'd read about in a magazine. They felt pretty sure this plan would work.

What's your health plan built out of? Quick-fix plans built out of panic or fear are easily blown down. But a well-thought-out plan built out of a strong desire can stand up to the huff and puff of temptation. Today marks the 18th day of your 30-day sugar-free commitment. You've proven you have staying power. Let's keep that momentum going strong.

Daily Action: Recognize Your New Healthy Habits

Today, I'd like you to acknowledge positive changes you feel you can continue following after *Zero Sugar / One Month*. For example:

- Have you discovered that eating a daily salad makes it easy to control hunger in the afternoon?
- Are you pleasantly surprised you now enjoy raw nuts as a snack?
- Do you find delaying breakfast to practice intermittent fasting an effective strategy?
- Have you found that sipping hot tea after dinner helps you comfortably avoid dessert?

Sit quietly and consider the positive changes you've noticed since going sugar-free. Use the space below to record healthy habits you feel comfortable continuing after completing your *Zero Sugar* month.

_____

_____

_____

_____

Daily Result and Reflections: You did it! Your body thanks you for your new healthy habits! Now go get that check mark!

Self-Reflection: Fear is a false motivator. There's no denying it can push you to act. However, it's also a negative emotion that leads to stress, self-criticism, and feeling overwhelmed. How have you been using fear to motivate change? Have you told yourself you'd better change or else fill in the blank (such as you'll get a disease, be forever lonely, never measure up)?

_____

_____

_____

_____

_____

_____

Fear isn't a success strategy. It might feel familiar and leave you with the sense it must work if it's gotten you this far. However, rather than helping you, it makes you feel anxious, limiting what you can achieve. By following *Zero Sugar / One Month*, you've acquired new skills, knowledge, and experience. It's been your hard work and commitment, not fear, that has made the difference.

DAY 19

ONE DAY AT A TIME

Daily Focus: Today, you build your awareness that the only way to win the race is to keep moving forward one step at a time.

Daily Motivation: *What One Day at a Time Really Looks Like* Once upon a time, there was a hare who boasted about how fast he was and relentlessly teased a tortoise for being so slow. Tortoise grew tired of the boasting and challenged Hare to a race. "Surely you must be joking," chuckled Hare. "There is no way you can win!"

The two agreed to the race, and at dawn the next morning, they stood at the starting line. At the sound of the gun, Hare was off like a light. He ran ahead until he came to a bend in the road, where he stopped to look back. When Hare saw how slowly Tortoise was moving, he paused to rest at the base of a tree. In such a relaxed state and so certain of his victory, Hare drifted off to sleep.

Tortoise continued to plod ahead, never stopping, moving slowly but continuously forward until he was nary a yard from the finish line. All the animals who had gathered started to cheer for Tortoise, which woke Hare from his sleep. Realizing what had happened, Hare leapt to his feet and ran with all his might toward the finish line, but before he could get there, Tortoise crossed the line, winning the race.

Okay, I know you've heard that story many times—and the moral is obvious: The one who wins is the one who keeps moving forward and doesn't stop. But the distractions of modern-day living make this sage advice easier said than done.

An unfortunate truth is that life won't calm down so you can concentrate on reaching your goal. In fact, it can sometimes feel like life is conspiring against you. Have you ever started on a plan and then come down with a cold or had some problem come up that demanded your attention? Most of us have and there are critical moments in life that require us to say "time-out." However, your ability to work through lesser distractions is determined not by the problem but by your mindset and commitment.

Goal-achievers understand that consistent effort and persistence win the race. However, that knowledge doesn't make them immune to discomfort. Growth isn't a comfortable thing and progress isn't always visible. But as long as you keep taking steps in the right direction, your goal will materialize.

Here's another truth: Time passes. Counting today, there are 12 more days to go to fulfill your *Zero Sugar / One Month* commitment. Regardless of what you do with those remaining days, they'll come and go. Yes, it's hard to change and giving up sugar is something many people aren't willing to do. Chances are, you have friends and family members who are moving through their days slurping down lattes and munching on whatever is put in front of them without a care. Today, it looks like they're winning and you're suffering needlessly. But that's today. Tomorrow is a different story. It doesn't matter who you are, you can't outrun the consequences of a sugar-filled diet. It's a significant factor in the onset of diabetes, heart disease, and many forms of cancer. It causes chronic inflammation, making simple tasks like walking painful, and it heightens anxiety and depression.

The discomfort you feel today will be offset tenfold in the years to come. Your efforts are making a difference. Because of your actions, your body is creating fat-burning enzymes, making you a more efficient fat-burner. Your taste buds and brain chemistry are resetting, making your once-irresistible sugar cravings more manageable. Because you're willing to do today what others aren't willing to, you get the privilege of living in a body that feels right and that's physically capable of letting you live the life you want to live. That doesn't just happen—it's earned.

Life will happen over the next 12 days. You might be attending a birthday party. You might have a big work deadline or have a disagreement that leaves you feeling shaken. You don't have to eat sugar. The choice is always yours and is yours to make daily.

Daily Action: Stay in Today

A common adage in recovery programs is "one day at a time." It's a reminder to deal with each day's challenges as they come and not worry about what tomorrow might bring. There's a lot of wisdom in this approach. When we look too far ahead or at the distance we still must travel to reach a goal, it invites overwhelming feelings. If we commit to nothing more than the next 24 hours instead, it doesn't eliminate challenges, but it feels more doable.

Today, you'll focus on what the day has in store and not worry about the future. When you notice your mind projecting into the future, trying to solve (or worry about) a future problem, remind yourself that today is the day that requires your attention. This will take practice and you'll lapse into future thinking at least a few times today. However, you'll also have moments when you successfully pull yourself back to the present, giving yourself a glimpse at just how much calmer and in control this simple shift makes you feel.

Daily Result and Reflections: You did it! Another day is in the books. Go get your "I Did It!" check mark!

Self-Reflection: When it comes to regaining your health or losing weight, you might feel like a tortoise in a world full of hares. Slow results can be frustrating, but remind yourself that consistent effort wins the race. Think back over your *Zero Sugar* journey and share any thoughts on how this one-day-at-a-time philosophy has benefitted you.

_____

_____

_____

_____

_____

_____

DAY 20

MAYBE I'M OKAY

Daily Focus: Your hard work is paying off! There's still work to be done, but for today, you are okay.

Daily Motivation: *Effort vs. Reward* Becoming a mom was a defining moment in my life. I realized immediately upon the birth of my daughter that motherhood wasn't just some project you take on for a while but rather a lifetime commitment. Of course, that was perfectly okay with me because the rewards greatly outweighed the effort.

Health is like parenthood in this way. True health isn't achieved by practicing healthy habits every once in a while—it takes consistent effort. At times, that effort is uncomfortable and inconvenient, but the rewards are too numerous to count.

And here's something you might not realize: By abstaining from sugar for the past 19 days, you've already moved the needle on sustainable health and weight control.

No longer does your metabolism primarily depend on glucose (sugar) from your diet. It can now run efficiently on fat—*from your diet or body*—and make its own glucose when needed (a function of your liver). This ability to switch from burning sugar to burning fat is known as being metabolically flexible. This flexibility gives you freedom. Common issues, such as fatigue, hunger, and cravings, no longer rule your life because your metabolic engine never runs out of fuel.

Yes, getting to this point took effort and your attention is still required to keep the benefits rolling. But the big challenge of making the transition is behind you. As Eoin discovered, the effort is real, but the rewards are immeasurable.

For Eoin, the first couple weeks without sugar were intense as he found himself dealing with psychological and emotional factors. He experienced inner feelings of emptiness that in the past would be quieted by reaching for something sugary. With sugary treats no longer an option, there was now nothing left to fill that void. The discomfort this created left him feeling scared and in something of a funk. However, these feelings passed and he now looks forward to a life without sugary processed foods. He feels like he's escaped the clutches of the devil and dodged the biggest bullet in the world.

Daily Action: Track Your Progress

For today's action step, you'll once again complete the self-evaluation to gauge your progress (pg. 126). However, I'd like to add an additional action step. As you go through your day, entertain the idea that you're doing just fine without sugar. And if you are okay today, you might just be okay keeping sugar out of your daily diet.

Daily Result and Reflections: You did it! Today's success means you're two-thirds of the way to the finish line. But who's counting? Another check mark awaits!

Self-Reflection: Today was a very special day. Statistics show that most people never see day 20 of their goal because day 19 is when most people abandon their efforts. You made it through the roughest of rough. Isn't that kind of cool? Use the space below to record your thoughts on reaching this stage of the game.

_____

_____

_____

_____

_____

_____

DAY 20 SELF-ASSESSMENT

Body Stats

Below, you'll find room to record your current body measurements. If you don't have access to all the measurements, simply record what you can.

Current Weight _____

Body Fat % _____

BMI _____

Fasting Blood Sugar _____

Measurements

Measure against bare skin. Use a flexible tape measure or a string you can later hold up to a ruler to determine your measurements.

Chest (measure around the fullest area) _____

Waist (measure one inch (2.5cm) above your belly button) _____

Hips (measure around the fullest area with your heels together) _____

Right Arm (measure around the fullest area above the elbow) _____

Right Thigh (measure around the fullest area) _____

Photos

Take selfies or ask a friend for help. Strike the same poses as you did on Day 0 (such as a full-body picture from the front, back, and side as well as a close-up of your face). For easy comparison, wear the same clothing for each photo session and stand in front of the same solid background.

Progress Chart

After filling in the Progress Chart below, compare your answers with those you gave on Day 0 (pg. 31) and Day 10 (pg. 81).

NON-SCALE ASSESSMENT	TRUE	MOSTLY TRUE	(UNSURE) NEUTRAL	MOSTLY UNTRUE	NOT TRUE
My pants fit loose.					
My rings fit loose.					
My sleep is restful.					
My ability to focus is strong.					
My energy level is high.					
My sugar cravings are low.					
My joints are pain-free.					
My ability to cope with stress is high.					
My outlook is positive.					
My nose is rarely stuffy.					
I do not snore at night.					
My skin is clear of blemishes.					
There is no swelling in my legs.					
My sense of accomplishment is high.					

DAYS 21-30

A Sneak Peek at the Key Points Ahead

Day 21: Comfort zones feel safe, but they limit opportunities.

Day 22: Enthusiasm builds when you lean into the feel-good truth.

Day 23: It's your unique strengths and talents that allow you to rise above the problem of sugar.

Day 24: Eliminating sweetness (not just sugar) locks in your results.

Day 25: Healthy foods become more appealing with sugar out of the picture.

Day 26: Rules provide the security needed to build confidence in your own decision-making abilities.

Day 27: All cravings pass.

Day 28: Happy things happen when you stop eating sugar (such as reduced weight, joint pain, cravings, inflammation, risk of diabetes, and much more).

Day 29: Easy to follow, enjoyable, and effective. When those three Es are in place, you'll have no need to return to old habits.

Day 30: You've reached your destination! Your body thanks you!

DAY 21

ESCAPING THE SUGAR COMFORT ZONE

Daily Focus: Comfort zones keep you stuck. Today, you are questioning your sugar comfort zone to pursue what you really want.

Daily Motivation: *Meet the Clampetts* You might have heard of a fictional television family known as the Beverly Hillbillies. They lived an impoverished life until the patriarch of the family, Jed Clampett, struck oil on his land.

I saw the script from one of their first shows. It was a conversation between Jed and Cousin Pearl that took place shortly after the oil discovery. At the time, he was still living on the outskirts of modern civilization.

Jed said: "What do you think, Pearl? You think I oughta move?"

Cousin Pearl replied: "Jed, how can you ask? Look around you. You live eight miles from your nearest neighbor. You're overrun with skunks, possums, coyotes, and bobcats. You use kerosene lamps for light. You cook on a wood stove, summer and winter. You're washin' with homemade lye soap. And your bathroom is 50 feet from the house. And you ask should I move?!?"

Jed thought for a moment and then responded: "Yeah, I reckon you're right. A man would be a dang fool to leave all of this."

Jed was stuck in his comfort zone. He was rich. But living poor. He had everything he needed to lead an easier life but couldn't embrace that abundance because it was too uncomfortable to change.

Zero Sugar / One Month requires you to step out of your sugar comfort zone. Before starting, you might have grown comfortable with a sugar-filled life, even if it had unwanted consequences. When you committed to 30 days without sugar, it was scary to think about getting through your afternoon without a syrupy sweet latte or spending the evening without ice cream. However, because of your commitment, you stepped out of your comfort zone and closed the door on those habits. While those treats might still sound good, consistent time away from them has turned what once felt like a need for sugar into somewhat of a calm indifference. (*"It would be fun to eat, but I'm okay without it."*)

Comfort zones take many forms—from daily treats to seasonal expectations. For example, the cooler fall temperatures scream at you to snuggle up with a cup of hot chocolate—and don't forget the marshmallows! Winter's dark skies invite nighttime snacks in front of the TV, spring brings Easter treats, and summer equals s'mores by the campfire. There's nothing wrong with enjoying life, but you want to set up safeguards so you don't fall back into a sugar-filled comfort zone.

Daily Action: Looking Ahead

Today's action step provides you with an opportunity to think about life beyond *Zero Sugar / One Month*.

We celebrate major holidays, birthdays, or life events every season of the year. We're blessed to be able to celebrate with food, but if these events are filled with sugary treats, they can feel like traps.

Below, you'll find a prompt for each of the four seasons asking you to write down an expected social event and a way to navigate through it without rejuvenating your sugar habit.

For example:

The winter event that comes to mind is Christmas.

To handle sugar, I can make and share Homemade Trail Mix (pg. 132).

To get into the right mindset, picture yourself at the event. Who's there that you enjoy spending time with? What nonfood activities are happening? What's available to eat that doesn't have sugar? If clear solutions for handling sugar at these special events don't come to you immediately, no worries. The remaining daily guides will get your creative juices flowing.

For now, simply posing the problem to your brain is enough to get it to search for answers. You might be surprised when one day, a solution pops into your head.

The winter event that comes to mind is _____.
To handle sugar, I can _____

_____

_____.

The spring event that comes to mind is _____.
To handle sugar, I can _____

_____

_____.

The summer event that comes to mind is _____.
To handle sugar, I can _____

_____

_____.

The fall event that comes to mind is _____.
To handle sugar, I can _____

_____

_____.

Daily Result and Reflections: You did it! Give yourself a big high-five and mark that report card!

Self-Reflection: Comfort zones are limiting. They make you feel as if there is only one way to make it through something, like thinking "*Surviving the afternoon requires a caramel mocha latte.*" When you let go of them, a world of possibilities opens up. If stepping away from your comfort zone feels uncomfortable, that's expected. Everyone experiences discomfort when changing their diet. Use the space below to reflect on a situation you handle differently today than before starting *Zero Sugar / One Month*. What benefits came from the change?

_____

_____

_____

_____

RECIPE FOR SUCCESS

HOMEMADE TRAIL MIX

Adults and kids will love this savory snack. Take it along on a trip, pack it in a lunchbox, share it in the office breakroom, or scoop it into glass Mason jars and give it away as a healthy holiday gift.

SERVES: 25 · **SERVING SIZE:** ABOUT ¼ CUP

1 cup (120g) raw whole almonds
1 cup (108g) raw sliced almonds
1 cup (140g) raw or dry-roasted peanuts
½ cup (55g) raw or dry-roasted macadamia nuts

½ cup (60g) lightly chopped raw walnuts
½ cup (60g) lightly chopped raw pecans
1 cup (118g) raw pumpkin seeds
1 cup (140g) raw sunflower seeds

FOR THE COATING

6 tbsp salted or unsalted butter
1 tbsp Worcestershire sauce
1½ tsp fine sea salt
1½ tsp chili powder
1¼ tsp onion powder

1¼ tsp garlic powder
⅛ tsp crushed red pepper
2 tsp Swerve Confectioners (found in most health food aisles or online)

FOR SERVING

¼ cup (35g) sugar-free chocolate chips (e.g., Lily's Semi-Sweet Style Baking Chips (optional)

1.   Preheat the oven to 300°F (150°C). Line two baking sheets with parchment paper. Set aside.

2.   Combine all the nuts and seeds in a large bowl. Set aside.

3.   Melt the butter and pour it into a large bowl. Add the Worcestershire, salt, chili powder, onion powder, garlic powder, red pepper, and Swerve sweetener. Whisk to fully combine.

4.   Add the nuts and seeds to the butter mixture and stir until the nuts are fully coated. Spread the mixture evenly between the two prepared baking sheets.

5.   Bake for 25–27 minutes, stirring every 10 minutes. Cool completely (at least 1 or 2 hours at room temp) before mixing in the chocolate chips (optional). Store in an airtight container for up to 2 weeks.

NUTRITION PER SERVING		
Calories 223	Carbohydrates 7.3g	Sugars 1.2g
Fat 20.6g	Fiber 3.6g	Protein 6.8g

"Enthusiasm won't stay alive without a positive focus."

LEAN INTO THE FEEL-GOOD TRUTH

Daily Focus: Just as a fire won't keep burning without more logs, enthusiasm won't stay alive without a positive focus. Today, you are stoking your inner fire by leaning into the feel-good truth.

Daily Motivation: *Feeding the Fire* I grew up in a one-story ranch home with a great fireplace. The earthy aroma and glowing embers filled the house with a peaceful ambiance. It was truly lovely. In the winter, we relied on the fireplace as our main source of heat. Before bed, Dad would turn down the electric heat and stoke the fire. It was so nice drifting off to sleep as the logs crackled and popped.

The serenity would end each morning because IT WAS COLD! So cold, in fact, that some mornings, you could see your breath. I quickly learned to remain sheltered under the blankets until I heard Dad feeding the fire, taking the chill out of the air. There was a simple truth hidden in those chilly mornings: If you don't keep feeding the fire, you'll grow cold.

Isn't this true of life? If you stop finding ways to feed your inner fire, the flame burns out and the cold seeps in. Enthusiasm is the name we give to that inner fire. It's the spark that makes us want to do things. If you want to follow a healthy lifestyle, you must feed your enthusiasm daily, including today.

Enthusiasm is more than a pep talk (although they have value). It's a by-product of your focus. For example, you can choose to focus on the things you can't do because of your *Zero Sugar* commitment or the things you're gaining from this experience. The first focus will leave you feeling grumpy and discouraged. The latter will build your motivation.

Notice that focus isn't about determining what's true about a situation. In fact, with *Zero Sugar / One Month*, two truths exist: You must give things up and you're gaining things. So focus isn't about finding "The Truth." It's about leaning into the truth that stokes your inner fire and makes you feel good. Doing so makes you much more likely to act in a way that agrees with your goal.

Daily Action: Lean Toward the Positive

Keeping your enthusiasm for healthy living strong is as easy as asking yourself the following questions.

What's one good thing that's resulted from not eating sugar for the past 21 days?

_____

_____

_____

_____

What about that makes me happy?

_____

_____

_____

_____

This might sound too simple to be effective, but you'll be surprised at how much leaning into the positive truth bumps up your enthusiasm level.

Tip Jar

Why not make this a daily enthusiasm habit? While you're still in bed in the morning or before you go to sleep at night, ask yourself: "What's one good thing that's coming into my life because of this sugar-free day?

Daily Result and Reflections: You did it! Flip back to your "I Did It!" report card, mark Day 22, and give yourself a well-deserved pat on the back.

Self-Reflection: Shifting your focus isn't about trying to convince yourself that one thought is more valid than another. You're simply leaning away from a thought that makes you feel bad toward one that makes you feel good.

Think back to a time when you were tempted to eat sugar. Notice how it was your thoughts about the situation, not the situation itself, that made it easy or hard to avoid eating sugar. (For example: A birthday party doesn't make you eat cake. It's your thoughts about what should happen at a party that makes it desirable.)

_____

_____

_____

_____

_____

"When the right thoughts are combined with the right actions, you're able to rise above the problem."

DAY 23

LIVING ABOVE SUGAR

Daily Focus: To live a sugar-free life, you must rise above sugar. The climb has challenges, but once you are perched on top, the problem is beneath you and manageable.

Daily Motivation: *Climbing the Ladder* To date, we've discussed the important role a positive mindset plays in living without sugar. That doesn't mean obtaining a sugar-free life is a simple matter of thinking happy thoughts. It also requires commitment and dedication. In other words, when the right thoughts are combined with the right actions, you're able to rise above the problem.

Imagine you're climbing a ladder. Let's suppose this is a metaphorical ladder of success. There are ladders for every area of life: finances, career, relationships, health, emotions, and social ladders. You've climbed these ladders all your life, overcoming obstacles and challenges as you ascend.

You climbed one of the first ladders when you learned to ride a bike. When you were in elementary school, Dad removed the training wheels and there before you stood a challenge. How in the world would you balance on only two wheels?!? You stood there at the bottom of the ladder, and for a time, the problem of learning to ride the bike was bigger than you. You felt scared and incapable of success. You feared what might happen if you tried and failed. Would you hit the pavement hard? Could you handle the pain of falling?

Then something happened—you heard Dad's encouraging words: "You can do it!" You saw the other kids successfully riding their bikes and having what looked like so much fun. You wanted to experience that fun, so you acted despite your fear. At first, it was hard. You didn't understand what to do and fear made you cautious. But soon, you moved a few feet on your own and you began to believe it was possible. Your small success gave you a glimpse of that joy and freedom your friends had, and although you'd inevitably fall, you got back up and tried again until that day came when you could hop on the bike and go without conscious thought.

That day, you took a step up on the ladder of success. You rose above the problem of riding a bike, and while it will always require some skill, riding a bike is manageable now because your thoughts about it have changed. Before you learned the skill, you thought riding a bike was nearly impossible. But by observing and modeling others, your desire, belief, and commitment grew, allowing you to see that riding a bike was not only possible but also easy!

When you focus on why a problem is too hard, you live below the problem. When you're below the problem, you look up and see an enormous obstacle and think it is too big, so you settle into life at the bottom of the ladder. You start to make up stories about why life at the bottom of the ladder is actually better. You tell yourself that those at the top of the ladder are just lucky—that they're blessed while you're cursed. You tell yourself you could do it too if you had their genes or their metabolism.

Before starting *Zero Sugar / One Month*, you stood on the bottom rung of the ladder leading to a sugar-free life. Above you loomed many obstacles and uncertainties, but you chose to start climbing. With each passing day, you strengthen your desire, belief, and commitment. The climb hasn't been easy. There were days when you felt you'd lost a step or two. However, you stuck with it, secured your grip on the next rung, and continued. This persistent effort is allowing you to rise above the problem. Perched on top of the ladder, you can look down and see that the mystery of handling sugar that once loomed heavy over your head is now beneath you and manageable.

Daily Action: Identify Your Strengths

To live a sugar-free life, you must rise above the problem of sugar. However, you might have past experiences that cause you to doubt your ability or leave you with a defeated mindset. The reality is you have everything you need to succeed. You just need to shine a light on those assets.

Overcoming sugar's pull has physical and mental components. Avoiding sugar—as you've been doing—allows you to tackle the physical factors. Today, you have an opportunity to highlight your internal strengths.

Below, you'll find a list of strengths and talents. Circle at least five that describe you.

adaptable	appreciative	articulate
athletic	capable	caring
clever	committed	compassionate
confident	consistent	courageous
creative	curious	determined
diligent	diplomatic	energetic
entertaining	enthusiastic	fair
fun	generous	grateful
hardworking	honest	humorous
imaginative	influential	insightful
intelligent	kind	levelheaded
logical	loving	open-minded
optimistic	organized	passionate
patient	perceptive	persistent
practical	reliable	resilient
resourceful	responsible	self-assured
self-reliant	sensitive	sincere
spiritual	strong-willed	supportive
thoughtful	trustworthy	understanding
versatile	willing	wise

By following *Zero Sugar / One Month*, you're accomplishing a lofty goal that's above the norm. Your success isn't some fluke or a lucky break. It's happening because of the unique strengths and talents you possess. You're making it happen.

Daily Result and Reflections: You did it! That report card is looking good!

Self-Reflection: Are you really missing out? Do you regret not eating sugar on Day 4? What about Day 12? Do you wish you'd eaten sugar on that day? Personally, I've never woken up and thought to myself, "Gee, I wish I'd eaten sugar yesterday." Below, record your response to this question: "Would this past month have been better if you'd eaten sugar?"

_____

_____

_____

_____

_____

_____

DAY 24

SHED THE CRUTCHES

Daily Focus: Today, your sugar-free transition takes flight with the elimination of excess sweetness.

Daily Motivation: *Do You Want a Ride?* I have the desire to fly an airplane. It's always interested me and I think I'm ready to go. Do you want to be my first passenger? Don't worry. I read a book on how the plane lifts off and what all the controls do. Now would you like to come along? Did I mention I interviewed a pilot? I picked his brain for nearly an hour and learned what to do if anything went wrong. I'm all set. Do you want a ride?

Hopefully, you see that taking me up on this offer wouldn't be a good decision. I certainly have an enthusiastic attitude about flying. I read and educated myself on how a plane works. But nobody in their right mind would go up in an airplane with me behind the controls until I turned this attitude and knowledge into action. It would take me many hours of supervised flight time to learn the intricacies of flying an airplane. Bottom line: There are things you can't learn from a book. Sometimes, you just have to do it to really get it.

Zero Sugar / One Month has allowed you to turn ideas into action. Your willingness to take action has moved you away from the addictive pull of sugary snacks and desserts. Today, you have an opportunity to lock in your results by distancing yourself from not only sugar but also sweetness. You'll do this by omitting sugar substitutes and limiting your fruit intake.

When you start a healthy eating plan, it's human nature to search for foods that act as substitutes for your old favorites yet technically fit the new diet's parameters. A common way to do this is to swap noncaloric sugar substitutes for sugar. The hope is that by eliminating the calories, you can continue to enjoy sweet treats without the consequences. However, the reward we experience when we eat something pleasurable is twofold, with sensory and postingestive (aka after-eating) components.

As you eat, the sensory branch is activated through taste receptors on your tongue as well as a part of your brain known as the "reward center" that responds to the sweet stimulus by releasing the feel-good chemical called dopamine.

The postingestive or after-eating branch has to do with the value your body receives from the food you ate. Satisfying this branch depends on the nutritional components of the food.

In other words, when you eat something sweet, you get sensory satisfaction because your taste buds and brain chemistry love it. But if that sweetness comes without nutritional value, the second branch of the food reward pathway goes unfulfilled, leaving you unsatisfied and looking for more to eat.

Zero-calorie sugar substitutes provide sweetness without nutritional value. They offer partial—but not complete—activation of the food reward pathways. The treat tastes good at the moment. However, by eating it, you've kept your sweet tooth alive so it can live another day and come back to bug you tomorrow. Angela discovered this when she stopped eating sugar but replaced it with an array of sugar alternatives, including stevia, allulose, monk fruit, and erythritol. She hoped the change was a healthy step in the right direction but found that consuming sugar substitutes kept her craving sweets.

Eliminating nonnutritive sweeteners makes sense, but why limit fruit? After all, fruit is packed with nutrients. It's true that fruit has fiber and other components that support the body and lock in the natural sugars, slowing digestion. These factors lessen the blood sugar and insulin spikes seen with the consumption of table sugar, reducing fat storage and dampening addictive factors. However, eating fruit throughout the day keeps your brain and taste buds hooked on sweetness, leaving the connection to sugar strong.

Tip Jar

Concerned about missing out on vitamins and minerals by cutting back on fruit? Don't be. Non-starchy vegetables contain plenty of vitamins and minerals. Replace fruit with a variety of vegetables and you won't miss a thing.

What about sugar substitutes with calories, like dried fruit, honey, agave, molasses, and maple syrup? These foods contain nutrients and natural fruit sugar, but the sugar has been concentrated, and with little or no fiber to slow absorption, these sweeteners fuel sugar cravings.

Daily Action: Eliminate Excess Sweetness

For this final week of *Zero Sugar / One Month*, I encourage you to omit noncaloric sweeteners, consume no more than two pieces of fruit per day, and omit concentrated sugar substitutes.

To clarify, here are the recommended rules for this final week:

- Omit all foods and drinks sweetened with a noncaloric sweetener. See a list of nonnutritive sugar substitutes in the FAQ section on page 18.

- Limit your fruit intake to two servings of fruit per day. You can choose any two whole fruit items. A serving is one medium-sized piece of fruit or ¾ cup (about the size of your fist) of smaller fruit, such as berries.

- Continue to avoid foods in which the natural fruit sugar has been concentrated. This includes dried fruit, honey, agave, molasses, and maple syrup.

Daily Result and Reflections: You did it! Another day in the bag!

Self-Reflection: Does avoiding excess sweetness feel empowering or intimidating? There's no right or wrong answer, so resist the urge to judge your answer as good or bad.

_____

_____

_____

_____

NEW WAYS TO MAKE FOOD CHOICES

Daily Focus: When sugar no longer dulls your senses and hijacks your brain chemistry, you are free to enjoy new flavors and effortlessly make better food choices.

Daily Motivation: *Taste Is Overrated* Yesterday, you kicked off the final week of *Zero Sugar* by further reducing your exposure to sweetness. By avoiding sugar substitutes and limiting fruit, you rise above the addictive pull of sugar, making it easier to make good food choices. Here's why: Choosing appropriate foods is an important part of leading a healthy lifestyle. Sugary drinks and refined carbs overload your brain and tastebuds, making sweetness feel like a necessity. In this overloaded state, you're prone to choose foods based almost entirely on one factor: taste.

Eating good-tasting food is pleasurable, but this desire for sensory gratification can override common sense. For example, if taste is the primary factor in determining what to eat, it's easy to eat too much. You can eat until you're stuffed and still eat a piece of chocolate cake because it looks too good to pass up. You can know that after eating that cake, you'll feel sick to your stomach and have to loosen your pants, but you just don't care because it tastes so good.

Those who achieve freedom from sugar recognize that taste is only one of the factors to consider when making food choices. They also take into account how hungry they are, which foods will help their bodies perform well and maintain a comfortable weight, which options will leave them feeling good, and which ones will satisfy hunger. They see food as an essential part of the big picture of well-being and their body as an instrument that, when cared for properly, can do what they want it to do.

These characteristics aren't reserved for those fortunate individuals who were seemingly born without a sweet tooth. A common phenomenon among those who abstain from sugar is that their taste for sugar changes, with many finding that sugar becomes too sweet to be enjoyable.

JC experienced this firsthand when she visited her mother's house for Christmas. It was her first Christmas sugar-free and she wanted to continue her new lifestyle. However, her mom made her favorite cookies. Her mother was 80 years old, and JC didn't want to hurt her feelings by not eating, so she told her she would sample them to let her know how they came out.

To her astonishment, she took one bite and the sweetness locked her up! She couldn't eat any more nor did she have the desire to. In the past, she could down three or four of the cookies in one sitting, but after being away from sugar, they tasted too sweet. That's when she realized she'd turned the corner.

Daily Action: Making Better Food Choices

Time away from sugar frees you up to make food choices based on criteria other than just taste. I enjoy many foods now that I found unappealing when I ate a high-sugar diet. A few that come to mind are avocados, Brussels sprouts, and sauerkraut. Back when the intense sweetness of sugar was overpowering my taste buds, I'd have never believed that one day, I'd voluntarily add these foods to my plate!

What food(s) do you enjoy now that you didn't enjoy before *Zero Sugar / One Month?* _____

_____

What do you enjoy about this food? _____
_____ (Insert any factor(s) that comes to mind or choose one from the list below.)

It tastes good.

It satisfies my hunger.

It helps me control my blood sugar.

It makes my stomach feel good.

It's full of nutrients.

Daily Result and Reflections: You did it! Another check mark awaits!

Self-Reflection: Spending time away from sugar quiets physical cravings. However, it's common to experience a lingering romanticism about eating it. To disconnect from those nostalgic thoughts, recall how you felt when you ate too much sugar in the past (bloated, gassy, tired, mentally foggy, etc.)

_____

_____

_____

_____

_____

_____

DAY 26

IS THAT THE FINISH LINE I SEE?

Daily Focus: Today, you are looking beyond the finish line, developing a "day-after" game plan.

Daily Motivation: *Handling the Day After* Is there anything better than seeing the finish line at the end of a journey? You've made it to Day 26 of your 30-day commitment. And yep, that finish line is in sight! Have you been making plans for Day 31?

You'll wake up that morning without the *Zero Sugar* rules governing your food choices. Today, I invite you to think about ways to handle your "day after." There are many ways to loosen the reins and still absolutely love eating without reinvigorating your sweet tooth.

Here are some suggestions for handling Day 31 and beyond:

Keep going! You've got the momentum rolling. Why not keep it going by sticking with the rules? The longer you go without sugar, the more you solidify the physical and mental changes. Need some guidance? Flip back to Day 1 and go for it!

Give yourself a non-food reward. We've been conditioned to think of food as a reward. But when you stop and think about it, you must admit it's a bit odd to celebrate breaking free from sugar by eating sugar. If you find yourself saying "Amen" to that thought, consider a nonfood reward for Day 31 and stay on track. Would a new pair of pants be fun to shop for now that you've lost weight? Is there an antique store or vintage clothing shop you'd like to visit? Give it some thought. You've got a few days to figure out that special something.

Pick one sweet or high-carb treat. Don't buy it yet—just mentally choose it. Got it? Great! Now stop picking to avoid choice overload. The phenomenon known as the "paradox of choice" shows us that having many options to choose from requires more effort and can leave you feeling unsatisfied with your choice. When you consider fewer options, you quickly evaluate the good and bad of the item, increasing satisfaction and eliminating "what ifs." When Day 31 comes, enjoy your treat and then get right back on track.

Eat a keto-friendly dessert. These modified desserts are high in fat and low in carbs, with a touch of sweetness. That combination does a better job of satisfying hunger and maintaining a stable blood sugar level than traditional desserts loaded with white flour and sugar. Allowing this non-sugar but still sweet treat will feel like a splurge with less worry of backsliding into your old sugar habit. Why not try my Raspberry Cheesecake Bites? You'll find the recipe on page 164.

Take one meal off. This can work because it feels freeing to eat whatever you want for an entire meal. The meal you choose is up to you. Does a big breakfast at your favorite restaurant sound good or would you rather stick to your no-sugar plan for the first part of the day and then relax the rules for dinner? The choice is yours.

Use intermittent fasting to your advantage. Instead of an entire day of splurging, split your day between a period of fasting and eating. For example, fast until noon, have a hearty salad for lunch, and go out for pasta for dinner. Shortening your eating window can naturally reduce your daily calorie intake, but know your limit. Pushing yourself to do an extended fast can backfire, making you too hungry to stay in control.

Eat more. Stick to your *Zero Sugar* pledge and splurge on larger than normal portions of lower-carb/better-carb, healthy-fat foods. In other words, have a high-calorie day but not a high-sugar day.

Abandon all rules. Day 31 is your free day, so there's no right or wrong way to go about it. If you decide to approach the day without any rules, go ahead, but pay attention to how you feel during and after your free day. There's a romanticism about the freedom to eat whatever you want. However, when you overindulge, you might see that freedom comes at a cost. That cost might present itself as unpleasant physical symptoms, such as a bloated stomach or urgent bathroom visits, or trigger cravings and mood swings that take time and effort to bring back under control—as Sonia experienced after being without sugar and refined carbs for 40 days.

Sonia saved her first day off for a work banquet right before Christmas. After being away from sugar and refined carbs for 40 days, she ate pasta and several bites of many types of desserts that were shared at her table. That night, she spent time in the bathroom with diarrhea and stomach cramps. The next morning, she woke up mad at the world, irritable, anxious, and just completely out of sorts. Her husband asked her what was wrong before she realized the impact sugar and refined carbs had on her health and mood.

The bottom line is that if you intentionally (or unintentionally) overdo it on Day 31, it can be a valuable learning experience. And you might just find that you felt so good without sugar that you can't wait to get back on track.

Daily Action: Pick Your Strategy

Now it's your turn. Look back over the suggestions for handling Day 31 and write down the strategy that feels right for you. Add any details that will help you bring that day into focus. Your approach can change over the remaining days of the program, but contemplating your choices now will help you make a smooth transition.

_____

_____

_____

_____

Daily Result and Reflections: You did it! That finish line is getting close!

Self-Reflection: Day 31 is a day without rules! That's good news, right? While it seems to go against common sense, many people find freedom when they have rules to follow. Rules feel safe and secure, providing a reason for our actions that doesn't have to be justified. "Why am I avoiding sugar? Because I'm following *Zero Sugar / One Month*." Use the space below to record how you're feeling about Day 31. Your future self will thank you for capturing your thoughts today.

_____

_____

_____

_____

DAY 27

YOU ARE BECOMING SUGAR-FREE

Daily Focus: One of the pleasant side effects of your consistent efforts is that sugar is no longer in control. You are becoming sugar-free, and it feels good!

Daily Motivation: *Losing Your Taste for Sugar* By now, you're in on the secret: To stop eating sugar, all you have to do is stop eating sugar. Yeah. I also think it's a cruel joke, but it's true. This is why having the structure of *Zero Sugar / One Month* is so valuable. It keeps you focused and on track long enough for your body and brain to accept the fact that all is well without sugar.

Yes, you still have thoughts about eating sugary treats. But sugar is no longer in control, making deciding what to put in your mouth easier. This is a big step toward becoming sugar-free and it's a proven phenomenon.

A study published in the January 2016 issue of *The American Journal of Clinical Nutrition* set out to determine what it took to diminish your taste for sugar. The participants were split into two groups. One of the groups was assigned to eat a low-sugar diet for three months, while the other group served as the control and didn't change their sugar intake.

Each month of the study, the participants were brought in, fed sweetened pudding, and asked to rate the sweetness of the treat. During the first month, both groups had equal ratings. But after that initial month, the low-sugar group rated the pudding samples as more intensely sweet than the control group. And this overly sweet perception grew as the low-sugar participants entered their third diet month.

What we can take away from this study is that you can train your taste buds to dislike intense sweetness, but to get there, you need to stay away from sugar for at least one month. This 30-day sugar-free period allows your body to make essential changes that prime it for easier health and weight control as time goes on.

Daily Action: Allow Cravings to Pass

It's empowering to know that because of your actions over the past weeks, your body has changed and you're becoming sugar-free. However, that doesn't make you immune to cravings. The important thing to understand is that all cravings pass. Whether you eat a sugary snack or not, that craving will go away. Trish found this to be true. Her secret for revamping her health, nutrition, and weight was to clear unhealthy foods out of her environment. She admits she still experiences occasional cravings. However, they pass as long as she's eating proper foods.

To complete today's action step, think back over your month and recall a time when you successfully waited out a craving. Think about your answers to the following questions.

- Were you saved from eating unhealthy food because there were no refined foods in your house?
- Did the treat not seem worth breaking your *Zero Sugar* commitment?
- Were you able to divert your attention to something else?
- Did you satisfy your hunger with a no-sugar meal?
- Did you use a Stopper?
- Did you call a friend or family member?
- Did you recall your "Big Why"?
- Did you figure out it was false hunger?
- Was it something else?

Use the space below to recall the experience and how you succeeded in staying on track with your *Zero Sugar* commitment.

_____

_____

_____

_____

_____

_____

Daily Result and Reflections: You did it! Another sugar-free day is in the bag!

Self-Reflection: A common observation of those who successfully break free from sugar is that their once-intense obsession with sugar has turned into a sense of calm indifference. Share your thoughts about this statement. Can you see how sticking with your *Zero Sugar* commitment might not eliminate cravings but can make them manageable?

_____

_____

_____

_____

_____

_____

DAY 28

COMPLETING THE JOURNEY

Daily Focus: You have come a long way, but 28 days are not the same as 30. Today, you choose to keep your eye on the prize, upholding your 30-day commitment.

Daily Motivation: *Are We There Yet?* A couple times a year, my husband and I pack up our vehicle and embark on a 1,300-mile trip to visit his mom. At times, the trip is fun as we experience the freedom of being out on the open road. Other times, it's boring as minutes drag into hours of nothing but highways. Those boring times make us question what we're doing and lament not having chosen a quicker mode of transportation. But there we are, stuck somewhere between "When will this end?' and "We're too far to turn back now." It's the classic "Are we there yet?" predicament.

When traveling to a destination, you can't just stop the car and declare you've gone far enough. However, with health goals … well, will one or two more days really make that much difference? In the grand scheme of things, maybe not. But I must attach a tough love warning: If you quit now, telling yourself that you're close enough, you'll regret it.

Regret is more than just a feeling. Research shows that when it's caused by inaction, regret is more likely to result in negative consequences, including stress, anxiety, and a feeling of being stuck. In other words, stopping now is problematic.

Today, I invite you to take in the big picture and relish what you've accomplished and what you'll continue to accomplish as you carry on with your sugar-free life.

Here are six happy things that happen when you stop eating sugar:

1. **Reduced Cravings** Avoiding sugar makes your brain and taste buds more sensitive to sugar, naturally reducing cravings.

2. **Reduced Inflammation** The most underrated precursor to poor health, inflammation is tied to many chronic disorders. Your commitment to no added sugar lowers your risk of high blood sugar, an inflammatory state.

3. **Long-Term Weight Control** Obesity rates are rising and sugar deserves a big chunk of the blame. Added sugar increases your calorie intake and stimulates your appetite. With it out of your diet, weight control is much easier.

4. **Reduced Risk of Diabetes** Type 2 diabetes is classified as a lifestyle disease, meaning the disorder is produced by or exacerbated by lifestyle choices, such as a poor diet and a lack of exercise. A hallmark of the condition is chronically high blood sugar levels. The best way to control high blood sugar is to not eat sugar.

5. **Fewer Cavities** I've often said that I was a sugar addict and have the cavities to prove it! For me, cavities are a thing of the past and they can also be for you now that you don't eat sugar.

6. **Less Joint Pain** When sugar is digested, it releases pro-inflammatory substances into your body, causing inflammation and pain in your joints. Cutting sugar not only gives you a healthier body, but it also improves your quality of life.

Daily Action: Identify What Healthy Means to You

Motivation is generated in two ways: We're either running away from something we don't want or running toward something we do want. The problem with running away is that it's rooted in fear, which builds anxiety. Today, you'll take the positive route, running toward your best life. Write down the long-term benefits you want that make it worth staying away from sugar. Use the word cloud below for ideas or add your own.

_____

_____

_____

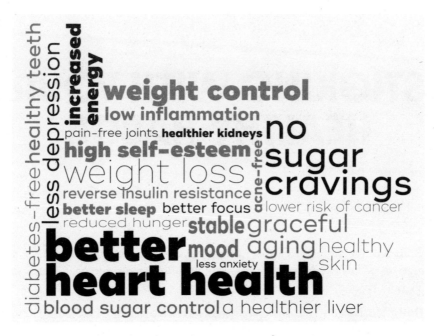

Daily Result and Reflections: You did it! Yes!!! This was a big day, so give yourself a great big smiley face or favorite mark on your "I Did It!" report card.

Self-Reflection: There are only a few days of *Zero Sugar / One Month* remaining. Do you feel it's worthwhile to stick with your *Zero Sugar* commitment and reach Day 30? Why or why not?

_____

_____

_____

_____

_____

_____

STICKING WITH YOUR HEALTHY HABITS

Daily Focus: Your hard work over the past month has set you up for a lifetime of healthy habits that are easy to follow, enjoyable, and effective. That feels good!

Daily Motivation: *You Are Three E Ready* Many years ago, I took a side job as a freelance science writer. I'd be assigned a health and nutrition topic, write a script, make an audio recording of what I wrote, and then hand my work over to a video editor, who would turn it into a wonderfully illustrated video that was used by high school and college students as an educational tool.

One of the topics I was assigned was to cover why so few people stick with healthy habits. Through my research, I came across a report in *Nutrition Today* magazine by a panel of doctors that truly changed the course of my teachings from that day forward.

The group discovered that the problem isn't that we don't know what to do. We all know we should exercise and not eat junk food or smoke cigarettes. But when we set out to make a change, we get confused by all the conflicting information that bombards us daily. We get facts from the health consultant on the morning talk show, catch the health minute on the radio as we commute to work, and hear from our coworker about their new diet we just simply must try.

With so much information, the reason we stay where we are is not that we don't know what to do—it's that we know too much and therefore suffer from information overload. That leaves us feeling overwhelmed and we stall before we even get started.

Fortunately, this panel didn't stop at identifying the problem. They also found the solution. They discovered that when a person's plan was simplified so it didn't take over their life, when what they were doing had an element of enjoyment to it so they didn't feel miserable every day, and when their plan provided clear evidence their efforts were working, they stuck with their plan and reached their goal.

In other words, they'd created a way of eating and moving that was easy to follow, enjoyable, and effective. Those are my three E's. They've become my foundation for healthy living, and because of your hard work over the past month, you've also tapped into them.

Let's look at how *Zero Sugar / One Month* has set you up for an effective, easy-to-follow, and enjoyable lifetime of healthy living.

Effective: It's hard to find anyone who doesn't know that eating a high-sugar diet is unhealthy. However, there's a big difference between knowing something and acting on it. This past month, you did what others weren't willing to do: You took action—and now you're reaping the rewards because of your effort.

Easy to Follow: "Easy to follow" is different from "easy." Our world doesn't make it easy to live a healthy life. In fact, quite the opposite is often more truthful: It's easy to lead an unhealthy life. However, you can't outrun the effects of a poor diet, so that easy life will eventually lead to a very difficult and painful one.

While a healthy life isn't easy, it can be easy to follow. But here again, there's some irony. Setting up a healthy, easy-to-follow lifestyle requires work. Fortunately, you've already done much of that work.

Take a look at your daily routine now compared with 29 days ago. I'm willing to bet you've created habits that are easy for you to follow and effective for keeping you on track. Maybe a big salad for lunch is your trick for avoiding the mid-afternoon munchies. Maybe sticking with low-carb/healthy-fat foods helps you feel in control of cravings. I totally understand that avoiding sugar doesn't mean you always feel like sticking with it, but because of your work, you can do it with less effort.

Enjoyable: Like "Easy to follow," enjoyable can be tricky. Sugar is a deceptive character. It gives you an immediate boost in energy and well-being but then robs you of those things, making you obsessively crave more. The more you eat, the more you need as your taste buds and brain chemistry dull to the intense sweetness.

One of the most common "aha" moments experienced by those who give up sugar is how much they enjoy the taste of healthy foods now that their physiology isn't hijacked by sugar. Can you see how this is true in your life? Can you taste the subtle, pleasant sweetness of natural foods, such as berries, nuts, and seeds? When you're free of the dominance of sugar, you discover that there's a whole world of flavors out there to enjoy!

Daily Action: Recognizing Your Three E's

Having the three E's in place doesn't remove temptation from your life but does give you a path to a healthy lifestyle. As you continue down that path, you'll reach milestones, gather favorite recipes, and feel better mentally and physically, which will have a snowball effect that makes it uncomfortable and undesirable to go back to your old habits. Reflect on how your habits have changed. What's something you routinely do now that's made healthy living easier to follow, more enjoyable, or more effective?

_____

_____

_____

_____

Daily Result and Reflections: You did it! One more day in the books—and one more to go! Wahoo!

Self-Reflection: Tomorrow is your last day of _Zero Sugar / One Month._ Answer these questions tonight to feel in control of tomorrow.

Is there an event tomorrow that will be serving sugar? If yes, how will you handle it?

_____

_____

_____

_____

_____

_____

What will you have for breakfast? _____

_____

What will you have for lunch? _____

_____

What will you have for dinner? _____

_____

Do you have the ingredients on hand to prepare your meals? _____

_____

DAY 30

YOU'VE ARRIVED AT YOUR DESTINATION!

Daily Focus: There is no more worthy pursuit than the pursuit of health. You have given yourself a wonderful gift, and there is so much freedom ahead because of your actions.

Daily Motivation: *Hello, Day 30!* Well, hello, Day 30! You can't believe how happy I am to finally meet you!

Yes, it's true. Day 30 has arrived. While you still have some hours to go to officially finish out the month, you should have a smile on your face.

Over the past 29 days, you chose commitment over convenience and blazed a path to better health that fits into your lifestyle without taking over your life. At times, you felt challenged; at others, hopeful and empowered. Admittedly, putting *Zero Sugar* into action required effort, but soon into this journey, the results started to show, proving that your perseverance was paying off.

Don't underestimate what you've accomplished. This wasn't just a one-month experiment. You proved you could take on a challenge without faltering, giving in, or making excuses. You put your money where your mouth is and stuck with it regardless of peer pressure and hard times when that little voice in your head tried to convince you that you'd come far enough. And now, here you are on Day 30! Excuses are easy but fill you with regret. Commitment is tough but fills you with pure joy! Well done!

Final Daily Action: View Your Results

For today's action step, you'll complete your final self-evaluation to reveal your results. You'll find the evaluation on page 165. However, I'm adding one last action step: Take time today to prepare for tomorrow (Day 31).

Tomorrow is indeed a day without rules, but it's also true you don't want to throw caution to the wind and slide back into old destructive habits. Why not make some healthy, no-sugar snacks to have on hand? Maybe restock your survival pack (page 57) or whip up some Raspberry Cheesecake Bites (page 164) to lessen the urge to go and buy sugary snacks.

I know. I know. It has been so long. But there's no shortage of refined foods. If you don't buy it today, it will still be on your grocer's shelf tomorrow. Have fun and enjoy the day, but don't make it easy to overindulge by restocking your snack food drawers.

Daily Result and Reflections: You did it! That final block on your "I Did It!" report card is going to feel so good to fill in.

Self-Reflection: The next time you find yourself in front of a mirror, look into your eyes, smile, and say "Good job." Even if you weren't perfect, you accomplished something exceptional. Your body is happy you took the time to care for it in this way and you'll reap the benefits. Congratulations!

Share any parting thoughts or just give yourself a big hug. You deserve it!

_____

_____

_____

_____

_____

_____

RASPBERRY CHEESECAKE BITES

With the whole-food sweetness of raspberries and the creaminess of cheesecake, this quick-to-make treat is yummy for all!

SERVES: 6 · **SERVING SIZE:** 1 CHEESECAKE BITE

---

18 raspberries
4 oz (112g) cream cheese
1 tbsp no-sugar-added almond butter

2 tbsp allulose (strongly recommended for its favorable freezing properties)
¼ cup (27g) raw sliced almonds

1. Place 1 raspberry in 6 of the cups of a silicone mini muffin tray.

2. In a medium bowl, combine the cream cheese, almond butter, allulose, and the remaining 12 raspberries. Use a hand-held mixer to blend until smooth.

3. Spoon the cream cheese mixture into a plastic bag, cut off a corner of the bag, and gently squeeze the mixture into each muffin cup, surrounding the raspberry.

4. The cheesecake bites will be served upside down. To create a smooth bottom, swipe a knife over each cup so the filling is flush with the top of the mold. Freeze for 1 hour.

5. While you wait, place the sliced almonds in a separate plastic bag. Use a kitchen mallet to break them into very small pieces. Place them on a small plate and set aside.

6. Pop the frozen cheesecake bites out of the tray and wait 5 minutes for the bites to soften slightly. Roll each one in the almonds. Serve right away or store them in the refrigerator for up to 1 week or freezer for up to 1 month. If frozen, defrost for 10 to 15 minutes before serving.

Notes:

The silicone mold makes for easy removal, but you can use a regular muffin pan or a truffle mold.

If you use a sweetener other than allulose, the treats will freeze solid. If frozen, defrost in the refrigerator for about 1 hour before serving.

You can use slivered or whole almonds that are broken into small pieces or lightly ground in a food processor. Substitute chopped pecans or walnuts.

NUTRITION PER SERVING		
Calories 113	Carbohydrates 5.6g	Sugars 3.9g
Fat 10.4g	Fiber 1.3g	Protein 3g

DAY 30 SELF-ASSESSMENT

Body Stats

Below, you'll find room to record your current body measurements. If you don't have access to all the measurements, simply record what you can.

Current Weight _____

Body Fat % _____

BMI _____

Fasting Blood Sugar _____

Measurements

Measure against bare skin. Use a flexible tape measure or a string you can later hold up to a ruler to determine your measurements.

Chest (measure around the fullest area) _____

Waist (measure one inch (2.5cm) above your belly button) _____

Hips (measure around the fullest area with your heels together) _____

Right Arm (measure around the fullest area above the elbow) _____

Right Thigh (measure around the fullest area) _____

Photos

It is time for your post-program photos! Aren't you glad you snapped your first set on Day 0? Take selfies or ask a friend for help. Strike the same poses as you did on Day 0 (such as a full-body picture from the front, back, and side as well as a close-up of your face). For easy comparison, wear the same clothing for each photo session and stand in front of the same solid background.

Progress Chart

After filling in the Progress Chart below, compare your answers with those you gave on Day 0 (pg. 31), Day 10 (pg. 81), and Day 20 (pg. 126).

NON-SCALE ASSESSMENT	TRUE	MOSTLY TRUE	(UNSURE) NEUTRAL	MOSTLY UNTRUE	NOT TRUE
My pants fit loose.					
My rings fit loose.					
My sleep is restful.					
My ability to focus is strong.					
My energy level is high.					
My sugar cravings are low.					
My joints are pain-free.					
My ability to cope with stress is high.					
My outlook is positive.					

NON-SCALE ASSESSMENT	TRUE	MOSTLY TRUE	(UNSURE) NEUTRAL	MOSTLY UNTRUE	NOT TRUE
My nose is rarely stuffy.					
I do not snore at night.					
My skin is clear of blemishes.					
There is no swelling in my legs.					
My sense of accomplishment is high.					

DAY 31 & BEYOND

MAINTAINING YOUR MOMENTUM

Did you wake up with a smile on your face today? Yep! You did it! You accomplished something millions of others want to do but are unwilling to do. Sure, the journey was not without its obstacles, irritations, and slip-ups. However, you took action and stuck with it. For that, you deserve a big high-five!

I want to provide an important word about Day 31. You may have a wonderful day that leaves you feeling in control and filled with the joy of accomplishing something big. Or you might go off the rails and overeat sugar.

You may plan on abstaining, having just one bite of this or one nibble of that, but then out of the blue—Whoa!—the sugar gremlins reemerge. okay. It happens. It's not fun, and it is easy to get down on yourself. Know that you are not a failure for still liking sugar. Even if the sugar treat doesn't taste the same as it once did, it's hard for your brain to forget about that grainy white stuff.

If sugar catches you off guard, here's a recovery plan:

Step 1: Realize that you ate sugar because you are human. Take a deep breath and regroup.

Step 2: Eat a good meal. You've gathered some favorite whole-food meal ideas over the past month, and your body is primed to run on those hearty foods. Remember that your body has changed, becoming more metabolically flexible (see Day 20, pg. 124). That means it can run equally well on sugar or fat. That sugar you ate will be burned up, and when it's gone, your metabolism will switch back to fat-burning mode as long as you stop eating sugar. Give yourself permission to fill up on whole foods that are low in carbs and high in hunger-satisfying fats and protein. The Food List on page 22 will give you ideas.

Step 3. Use a Stopper. Even if you are full after your meal, that sugar gremlin might be whispering in your ear. Scoot him out of the way by using a Stopper. See Day 7 (pg. 66) if you need a memory jogger.

Step 4: Move on. Maybe you did not have your best moment; acceptance and moving on end the issue. Dwelling on it keeps you stuck.

WHERE TO FROM HERE?

The *Zero Sugar* experience is a unique opportunity to see sugar for what it truly is. It is a deceptive character promising fun and energy, then stealing those things from you and messing with your mood, focus, and hunger control. You don't want to be pulled back into its grasp, but you want to enjoy life. The solution is to do what is doable and avoid the mental and physiological triggers that nudge you back to your old ways. The more separation you create, the less sugar affects you, and the easier it is to hold on to this new lifestyle.

Individuals' food preferences, social demands, and daily activities vary. Therefore, what is doable for you and what triggers your desire to eat is unique to you. Below is a quick reference guide for building an easy-to-follow, enjoyable, and effective sugar-free life. It will act as a reminder without having to go back through the book.

Make sugar special, not ordinary.

How do you solve a problem like sugar? Its negative impact on health and well-being is evident, yet it is everywhere and, for the most part, socially accepted. Drawing a line in the sand and declaring that you will never eat sugar again will work for some. For others, that thought creates anxiety and fear that leads them right back into sugar's comforting arms. There's a middle ground: make sugar special, not ordinary. For example, a cupcake on your birthday is special. A cupcake in the breakroom is ordinary.

Don't allow yourself to get too hungry.

Having access to food is a blessing. However, past experiences and conflicting information can make it hard, even scary, to make food choices. This decision paralysis may lead to undereating that drives cravings. To feel good about your food choices, remember that whole foods are your friends.

Eat whole foods.

Whole foods are foods that you look at and recognize as something that exists in nature. They have been minimally processed with few, if any, ingredients added to them. Whole foods include meat, fish, eggs, nuts, seeds, fruits, vegetables, and legumes. Turn back to page 22 for a full list of food choices.

Experiment with carbs.

Through *Zero Sugar / One Month*, you discovered that not all carbs are created equal. Some trigger cravings and others don't. The more refined the carb, the quicker it is absorbed and the more you want to eat. Therefore, pancakes, muffins, white bread, and other highly-refined foods can be just as addictive as table sugar and should be avoided or reserved for special occasions. However, what about starchy vegetables (such as potatoes and corn), less processed grains (such as oats, sprouted-grain bread, and rice), natural sugars from fruit, honey, and dried fruit, or sugar substitutes like stevia and monk fruit? Whether or not these foods trigger cravings varies among individuals, so if you're interested in reintroducing them into your diet, do so one food at a time and note how you feel. For example, keep the rest of your foods *Zero Sugar* compliant, but add honey to your morning cup of tea and then evaluate how it affects your mood, energy level, and cravings throughout the day.

Be ready.

Life is full of surprises! Be ready by always having a Stopper on hand (sugar-free gum and dental floss travel well). Have healthy snack alternatives nearby (see Day 4, pg. 55). And, be "No thank you" ready ("No thank you, but I'd love a glass of water"), and you'll sail through any situation unscathed.

Have a "Big WHY."

The tips above share the how-to's for living a sugar-free life. However, knowing how to do something is of little value without a compelling reason for doing it. The Big WHY you came up with on Day 5 (pg. 59) may need to be expanded upon as you move beyond the program. Take a step back and consider what you really want from life. Not what you think you should want or what others view as correct. What do you want? You may discover that it is something big, like avoiding disease. However, in my experience, it is the little moments of life that make the effort worthwhile. It's that inner feeling of contentment when you like how you look in a photo. It's the ability to jog to your car when a thunderstorm pops up unexpectedly or get down on the floor to play with a grandchild—and get back up again—that counts.

And remember, you are a *Zero Sugar / One Month* alumnus, not because you got lucky or have ultra-human levels of willpower. Luck and willpower play a role, but they are fragile and unpredictable. You reached this point because you are strong and capable. It is those qualities that pave the way for a healthy life. You made it happen, and you'll continue to make it happen.

INDEX

ACKNOWLEDGMENTS

This is the book I have always wanted to write. So many of us want to live a healthy life but have no practical way of overcoming the hurdles that stand in our way. This book is about clearing those hurdles.

I want to thank Mike Sanders and the team at DK Publishing for believing in me enough to take on this project. A big thanks goes out to Brandon Buechley, who served not only as my editor but also as a sounding board and cheerleader for my ideas. From our first meeting, I knew I had an ally in this process.

Seeing my second book published fills me with joy. Yet, bringing a book through all the phases, from concept to publication, is, at times, all-consuming. This requires the support and understanding that only family can provide. And so, it is my husband, Keith, and daughter, Kelly, above all, whom I want to thank. They always manage to make me laugh and know just what to say to keep me from taking myself too seriously.

ABOUT THE AUTHOR

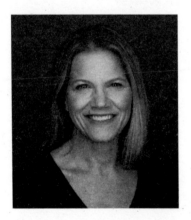

Becky Gillaspy, DC, is the creator of DrBeckyFitness.com. Her two YouTube channels, Dr. Becky Gillaspy and 2 Fit Docs (co-starring her husband Dr. Keith Gillaspy), together have garnered millions of views. Dr. Becky graduated summa cum laude with research honors from Palmer College of Chiropractic in 1991. She has worked as an on-air health consultant for a local ABC TV affiliate and spent most of her professional career teaching a range of college courses, from anatomy to nutrition. She is also the author of *Intermittent Fasting Diet Guide and Cookbook*.